Learning for Health Improvement

Learning for Health Improvement

A practical guide for the workplace

Lynne Caley MA, MA(Ed), D Phil
Director
Consolidated Caley Ltd

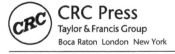
CRC Press
Taylor & Francis Group
Boca Raton London New York

CRC Press is an imprint of the
Taylor & Francis Group, an **informa** business

First published 2006 by Radcliffe Publishing

Published 2018 by CRC Press
Taylor & Francis Group
6000 Broken Sound Parkway NW, Suite 300
Boca Raton, FL 33487-2742

CRC Press is an imprint of Taylor & Francis Group, an Informa business

No claim to original U.S. Government works

ISBN-13: 978-1-84619-027-8 (pbk)

Visit the Taylor & Francis Web site at
http://www.taylorandfrancis.com

and the CRC Press Web site at
http://www.crcpress.com

Lynne Caley has asserted her right under the Copyright, Designs and Patents Act 1998 to be identified as author of this work.

British Library Cataloguing in Publication Data

A catalogue record for this book is available from the British Library.

Typeset by Anne Joshua & Associates, Oxford

Contents

Preface

Since the first NHS Plan was published in 2000, there has been a steady build-up in momentum towards change. We have seen efforts to increase capacity, to deliver some early reforms and to make step-changes in performance to improve services and reduce waiting times. At the same time there has been a move towards greater emphasis on clinical governance – a desire to improve standards and to secure patient safety. In aggregate we have seen improvements in the quality as well as the quantity of services offered. This is very good news.

However, significant as those changes have been, they are as nothing compared to the implications of the 'choice' agenda that lies just around the corner. The goal for the next few years is to deliver changes that are profound. Having reached this stage in modernisation of the service, the Government's stated policy is now to re-focus the whole system towards more choice, more personalised care, and real empowerment of people to improve their health. This mandate will require a fundamental change in the relationship between staff working in the service and the patient and service user.

We don't need a crystal ball to see that this will affect service delivery. Where, how and by whom care will be delivered will alter acutely. New and different organisational configurations will appear, and staff who have spent their professional careers working for the large bureaucracy that is the NHS may well find themselves working in radically new configurations in the private or not-for-profit sectors. The consequences of this could surprise many. There are subtleties of culture and behaviour that impact on everyday performance when a shift is made from one organisational structure to another. Staff need to be prepared for this. And service users who have been accustomed to a system that favours the passive consumer of healthcare may find it hard to manoeuvre their way actively through new and different routes to care.

All of those concerned will have to cope, and the way in which they will do so will be by *learning*. Some staff and patients will do this intuitively, because they are by nature adaptable and welcome change. Others will do it very reluctantly, or not at all. Of course staff can leave the service if they are unhappy with the new ways of doing things. But what about patients, particularly those who can't or won't exercise choice? How will they cope? They will need support to understand the reality of what is happening, and to make appropriate and effective choices. They need to *learn* how to interact differently with professional staff, who in turn need to *learn* how to interact with the new social environment that they inhabit.

Where did this kind of workplace learning come from and where is it going? My involvement in all of this stems from my personal and professional development as a health worker, an educator and a learner. I have seen the health service go through endless changes over the 30 or so years for which I have been involved with it – as a patient, as a worker, and as a supporter and adviser. I've worked in a sufficient range of workplaces, and witnessed the influence of social and cultural interactions, to see how they impact on getting the job done. I know from personal experience how exciting it is to learn new ways of doing things, and to create new ideas and see them make a difference to people's lives.

I first became interested in workplace learning when I was involved in the development of formal learning courses at a university. I could see the gulf between what was learned in the classroom and its application in the workplace. I began to construct courses that attempted to bridge this gap, and that drew on the experience of the workers/learners whom I supported. I started to realise that much useful learning took place in workplaces but was not recognised as such, and that some workplaces were better than others at encouraging learning and the sharing of learning.

Supporting workplace learning is never easy because it cannot be done in isolation from other workplace activities such as making widgets or providing a service. If the entire context of the workplace is under constant change, this can either enhance learning or condemn it to the sidelines. Which is it to be? I believe that change is exciting and provides fertile ground for creativity and innovation. I hope that this book will demonstrate to you that workplace learning will enable our shared ambition for a first-class health service to become a reality.

Lynne Caley
January 2006

About the author

Lynne Caley is an experienced senior consultant and manager who specialises in formal and non-formal learning for the benefit of individuals and organisations. She has had significant experience of working with organisations in the public and private sectors to develop and implement strategies for delivering high-level business outcomes, and she has extensive and specific knowledge of the NHS. As an outcome of her research Lynne has developed innovative methodologies and approaches derived from data and evidence gathering. She has successfully implemented and embedded innovative learning interventions, designed to lead to organisational change, in workplaces for teams of five to 500 people. After working at the University of Cambridge for many years, Lynne worked for the National Health Service University for the two years of its existence. She now acts as an independent consultant to education and healthcare organisations.

Acknowledgements

This book has been in gestation for a number of years, and is the result of much collaborative effort. I am grateful to a large number of people who, in conversations, workshops and workplaces, have shared with me their thoughts and ideas about workplace learning. The exercises and models that I have used were introduced to, and refined with, many managers from the NHS and social care who kindly gave up their time to work with me. I would like to thank them all, and also Elaine Hendry, Stuart Reid, Jake Reynolds, Chris Jude, Amanda Bassett and Maureen Murfin – friends and colleagues from my own workplaces. I would particularly like to thank Michael Eraut and Phil Candy, who have both made significant contributions to the field of workplace learning research, and who are my intellectual gurus. Finally, I would like to thank my husband Ray, who encouraged me to write this book.

For Ray, without whom this book would not have been possible.

Chapter 1

Introduction

Over the last decade there has been a big increase in the use of knowledge in all sectors of the economy in the UK, as well as in other parts of the developed world. You may have noticed that every job now has a 'skills profile' that is necessary to do the job (the Knowledge and Skills Framework is just one manifestation of this), and the vast majority of jobs require qualifications that are current and continuously refreshed. To a large extent this has been brought on by competitive pressures and new economic conditions. For example, we have seen the displacement of manufacturing to the Far East and other corners of the world. If you look at the label on almost any of your consumer goods – from shoes to clothes to washing machine – you will probably find that they were made in China, Brazil or somewhere else equally remote. The service sector shows the same pattern – the model of offshore subcontracting means that your telephone call to your bank might well be routed to India. To remain competitive in this globalised world, we here in the UK have to be more knowledgeable, more creative and more innovative than our peers abroad. As with other industries, this affects public-sector healthcare, where we have seen rising expectations on the part of service users, and drives for efficiency via published targets, all of which require increased knowledge.

Workers today need knowledge that is high in 'use' value which is specific to their work function, and which is short-lived, taking account of the dynamic nature of modern workplaces. In this book I shall argue that this kind of knowledge is developed collaboratively at work. Knowledge work and innovation emphasises the practical, and is interdisciplinary (i.e. not confined to one section of the workforce, but inclusive of all workers, whatever their background), contextual (i.e. influenced by the environment of the workplace) and procedural (i.e. concerned with processes and procedures). However, workplaces can be incoherent, can lack a structure to support learning and can have outcomes that are wholly specific to the particular enterprise involved. The question of how we deal with this forms the context for this book.

Coping with change

The UK Government regularly publishes policy documents designed to foster modernisation of the delivery of healthcare. Recent examples from the Department of Health (DH) include the *NHS Plan*; the *NHS Improvement Plan*; *Agenda for Change*; *Improving Working Lives*; *Practice Plus*; and *National Standards, Local Action: Health and Social Care Standards and Planning Framework 2005/06–2007/08*. Examples from the Department for Education and Skills (DfES) include a *Skills Strategy* and a *Skills for Life Strategy*; and examples from the Learning and Skills Council (LSC) include *Success for All, Equality and Diversity* and *Workplace Strategies*. All of these policy and strategy documents assume that change can't happen unless it is accompanied by learning.

To take just one example, the *NHS Improvement Plan* (published in 2004) emphasises *choice*, and it says that care should be responsive, convenient and based entirely around the patient and his or her individual needs. Choice in this context is not simply a matter of which hospital a patient might favour, but also includes the standard and focus of care that they receive when they get there. The underlying assumption is that patients will follow published information about where the best service is being provided. Therefore service users need to be well informed about these matters. But to respond to these new imperatives staff also need to be well informed, motivated and educated in all aspects of service delivery. They need to feel valued by their organisation if they are to continually improve on the service that they are providing.

More recently, the public health White Paper *Choosing Health: Making Healthy Choices Easier* (published in December 2004) set out the Department of Health's focus and aims for public health over the next four or five years. Clear priorities are the personalisation of services to patients and service users, with particular emphasis on priority areas for the health of the public, alongside consideration of long-term employment conditions in the service. New roles, such as that of 'Health Trainer', are to be developed, with the intention of enabling users of the service to take control of their own health priorities. This is about staff and service users undertaking learning together to improve the health of the community.

It's probably true to say that the NHS organisations within which we will be working in five years' time will bear little relation to the service we have today. We need to prepare for this, so that improvement can be ongoing and an integral part of everything that we do.

Change of this magnitude requires careful management and support of staff at all levels in the service. Middle and supervisory managers are pivotal in ensuring that staff develop the new skills and attitudes which are needed to effect these changes, and that they are enabled to use their new skills effectively. Supervisory managers are themselves learning, and they also need support. This kind of learning is most effective when it takes place alongside working, in the workplace, among like-minded people who are prepared to share their knowledge with others, so that everyone benefits.

With the growing pressure on the NHS to keep staff up to date, equipped with flexible and adaptable skills profiles, and with commitment to make a contribution over the long term, it is becoming necessary to look for creative ways to invest in people development. However, if this is confined to conventional solutions – taking people away from the workplace and sending them on training courses – the costs in financial and productivity terms will become increasingly prohibitive.

If our starting point is that work provides a basis for learning, this has significant implications for how we manage the worker/learner. We are concerned with outcomes that relate to performance – that is, behaviour – as well as with those that relate to knowledge and skill, important as they are. The workplace becomes the setting for learning and everyone present has a role to play. However, the success of this kind of learning rests significantly with one person, namely the supervisory manager, who sets the tone and manages the unfolding of the workplace as a site for learning.

Why is learning important for the NHS?

Since its inception in 1946 the NHS has been in a state of constant change, and the signs are that this will continue. Upheavals that have their roots in economic, political, demographic and technological circumstances have been a constant part of the experience of working within the ever-changing health and social care environment. For example, think about the following.

- Distance isn't what it used to be. Globalisation means that goods and services can be sourced from anywhere. Jobs are available on a world stage, so recruitment and retention of staff are made more difficult because experienced professionals are in demand everywhere and they can go anywhere.
- We're all living longer, and our expectations about our quality of life have increased so that the costs associated with providing healthcare have snowballed. At the same time, we aren't reproducing at the same rate. Families are smaller and the balance of old to young is shifting. It is predicted that by 2010 around 50% of the UK population will be of pensionable age.
- We live in a 'connected' world. The advent and spread of technology mean that we are all better informed and more demanding of the service that we are offered.

All of this adds up to a feeling of uncertainty and inadequacy among staff as they grapple with the pressures that are placed on them. End users witness a health service in turmoil. There are enormous issues surrounding recruitment and retention, resource allocation and planning, and these all impact on day-to-day performance.

Part of the response to these changes has been an increased emphasis on governance and clinical quality to improve patient care, over and above the everyday concerns of efficient management. These have been fundamental drivers of the current reforms, and their influence on the cost and delivery of healthcare has been profound.

Debate about ways to increase resources for the NHS is partly, but not entirely, economic. People's values are a critical part of the debate, and it is possible to detect strong associations between these and the reforms that have been recommended. Expansion (such as was outlined in the *NHS Plan*) undoubtedly requires more resourcing, but modernisation also needs more qualified, better skilled and more flexible workers. All NHS staff need to engage with learning as a priority so that these drivers (quality, efficiency, governance and patient care) are adequately understood and adhered to.

The promotion of improvement in the quality of service provided by the NHS and social care is dependent on a range of financial, cultural and psychological factors. The end result is a better patient/user experience, and this is achieved through developing a more skilled, reflective and effective staff, who are committed to the concept of lifelong learning.

The NHS has always recognised and emphasised the value of effective work-related learning, and this has required considerable ongoing resourcing and expenditure. Underlying assumptions about *how people learn while working* and how they can be helped to maximise their opportunities have perhaps been given less attention. Workplaces as learning environments differ, and these differences affect the amount and quality of learning that takes place. People learn in a variety of ways, with differences in approach and motivation. Attention needs to be given to these issues so that the best possible learning outcome is achieved.

What is work-related learning?

An efficient and cost-effective approach to these issues is to use the workplace and working activity as a site for learning. However, the term 'work-related learning' means different things to different people, and although there has always been a strong link between experience at work and the development of practical skills, there is still confusion about how work-related learning can best be managed. In this book I want to demonstrate that work-related learning can be much broader than mere skills acquisition, and that it involves not just the learner, but everyone in the organisation. In addition, the location of learning – the workplace – crucially influences how much learning takes place, and what and when learning will happen. Attention to the factors that influence learning will result in better outcomes for the learner, for their peers and for the organisation as a whole.

> Workplaces become what they are because of the systems that their managers design, the actions that they take, and the way in which they deal with risk. To cope with variation and ongoing change, workers need to learn continually – but so do managers.

Work-related learning is not a new idea. It's worth bearing in mind that the old craft apprenticeships such as plumbing and carpentry were once significantly work-centred, and this approach to skills acquisition was very successful for some workers in some craft industries. However, the training offered via conventional apprenticeships was not consistent, and there was an element of time-serving involved in many apprentice schemes. The need to provide more structure and consistency of experience resulted in a move away from workplaces into classrooms. Now we are witnessing a backlash, as it has become clear that theory alone will not make a good plumber, and that performance depends on having practical understanding which is best acquired through work. We now have 'modern apprenticeships' that don't much resemble those of previous generations, providing structured, relevant and innovative work-based learning opportunities.

Equally, the professions such as law and medicine have always relied on a version of work-related learning to supplement their formal degree process. However, the approach to learning employed by professional bodies has moved on since the days of hierarchy and restrictive practices. Some jobs (management springs to mind) have traditionally assumed that the skills necessary to perform well at work are best gained through experience, and jobs that provide challenge are the finest form of development available. However, the focus has shifted from an ad-hoc work-focused model which assumed that managing was intuitive and did not require any intervention to promote learning, to one involving structured learning that is delivered in a range of ways. In fact the range and number of learning opportunities are so great that confusion and uncertainty are apparent among those who commission learning and those who support it.

> It's worth remembering that:
>
> - **learning** is the process whereby a person constructs new knowledge, skills and capabilities
> - **training** is a method of promoting learning
> - **instruction** is one (but only one) of many techniques available to the trainer.

So although the concept of work-related learning is not new, what is emerging is a recognition that it should no longer apply to a minority of the workforce, but should be encouraged for all. We are beginning to realise that work-related learning offers relevant opportunities to share and to develop greater understanding of the reality of the way that the job is and can be done, alongside colleagues and workmates. Learning at and through work can increase job satisfaction and can enable people to perform more effectively. And the range of learning opportunities is growing.

How can we encourage work-related learning?

Universities apart, organisations are not set up primarily for learning. The NHS exists to provide a service to patients, and this activity remains the first priority for everyone working within the system. Learning in order to support this activity is certainly important, but it will always be secondary. This is not to say that learning cannot be maximised alongside the main functions with which the NHS is concerned.

The emphasis and energy given to learning will vary from sector to sector within the economy, and this will also alter over time. For most of the last century, the UK was a great manufacturing nation, with many men trained in skills for heavy industrial work, such as mining and shipbuilding, but there is no longer a call for such skills, as we now purchase our coal and ships from elsewhere. Where and what we call 'skills', and which are required, have all moved on, so it's true to say that the UK now needs a new kind of skill and a new kind of workforce. When we use the term 'skill' it's worth reflecting on how our definition has changed. Skill used to mean being able to change a washer or rivet a ship, but now it refers to something less tangible, closer to what we might call 'personal attributes', such as customer care, teamworking or interpersonal understanding.

As the general level of knowledge requirements has increased, so has the necessary sophistication of skills. 'Skills for life' include basic literacy, numeracy and IT, and these form the minimum requirements necessary in order to function in the modern world. A wide range of other skills have become necessary, the most significant of which are the skills of 'learning to learn' and 'information literacy'.

Although ideas about lifelong learning began to be spread in the 1960s, as late as the 1980s it was generally assumed that for the majority of workers all 'work-necessary learning' took place before the age of 21, and was sufficient to carry them through to retirement. We now recognise that our skill-set must change regularly, and that we have to continue to learn in order to keep abreast of the constantly changing world which we inhabit.

So if we are serious about the need to support work-related learning, we must first be clear about why people should learn, understand how people learn, and identify what they should learn, in order to improve their performance and thus improve the healthcare that they are providing. And we have to acknowledge the influence of the workplace and its occupants on the capacity of workers to learn. No one learns in isolation. Learning has a purpose, and that purpose is innovation and improvement, which can only be achieved as a group effort.

The significance of the environment for learning

For an organisation, the difficulty with workplace learning is managing what will be learned and how it can be harnessed. The manner in which organisations structure themselves makes them act in different ways. Some look like a machine with targets and indicators, somewhat like an assembly line, in which case the focus is on inputs and outputs, and people take second place. Others may mirror a community that is caring and alert for every member, where people are primarily there to assist each other in performing well, and outputs are the result of a shared endeavour.

If we look at organisations as the latter – as social systems within which people function – the emphasis is on the need to collaborate and participate within a group. Teams become a way of passing on shared understanding. In general I will argue here that an organisation which is bent on achieving improvement needs to go about it by encouraging learning, and it needs to focus not just on the circumstances that make learning necessary, but on its own systems and structures that either do or do not support learning, as well as the culture within which learning is embedded. A great deal has been written about organisations and change, and most of it is written in such a way as to suggest that change is non-problematic. In this book I shall look critically at these ideas, particularly with regard to the necessity and form of team structures and the sharing of ideas within organisations. The environment within the workplace is crucial for the success or failure of supportive learning.

> Workplaces are not set up for learning – they are there to make something or to provide a service, so learning will always take second place. However, that does not rule out the possibility of useful workplace learning. Whether the workplace helps or hinders learning depends on the people and the systems that are in place. Effectiveness can be achieved by paying attention to these factors.

Summary

It's true to say that the entire agenda of learning that relates to work has changed. We are now required to learn continually, both as individuals and as part of a group located within an organisation. Learning is no longer the personal concern of each member of the group, but is the joint and shared responsibility of all, and its purpose is to benefit organisational as well as personal growth.

In order to make sense of the complexity faced by the NHS as an organisation, an employer and a learning environment, we need to pay attention to the extent to which learning can be fitted alongside the provision of a first-rate health service. If we can agree on what helps and what hinders, we will be in a position to judge how close to an ideal we might be. We can then celebrate our strengths and focus on improving the weaker elements.

From the current literature emanating from the Government and the media it appears that the main drivers influencing the attention given to work-related learning for healthcare workers include the following:

- the *efficiency* with which the service can be provided
- the degree to which *accountability* within roles and responsibilities can be maintained during times of economic, social and technological change
- the level of *job satisfaction* within changing roles of healthcare workers
- the *quality of the patient experience*.

The effectiveness of the workplace as a site of learning is undoubtedly influenced by a number of factors. We need a way of recognising what those factors are to provide us with a framework for scrutiny and development. That is the purpose of this book.

The book is divided into 11 chapters. In this first chapter I have provided some background to the debate, and Chapters 2 and 3 explore a variety of theories about how people learn. I shall argue that work-related learning to promote health improvement is best described as collaborative and based around ideas of community. Chapters 4 and 5 consider the supervisory manager as a supporter of learning and locate him or her within the workplace environment, including an examination of some of the dilemmas that supervisory managers face in their role of supporting others. The supervisory manager is then placed within a broader NHS context in Chapters 6 and 7. Chapters 8 to 10 include a closer examination of the workplace itself and describe the organisational context within which learning occurs. A means of auditing the workplace to discover its strengths and weaknesses is also suggested. Chapter 11 then draws conclusions and lessons from all of this, and suggests the way ahead to improve patient care through work-related learning. At the end of each chapter there are suggestions for further reading and other resources of value to supervisory managers.

I hope that this resource book will prompt thinking and discussion about the vital issues that impact on learning in the workplace. You may wish to share your thoughts and ideas with others who have an interest in supporting workplace learning. There are a number of ways in which this can be done, ranging from conventional groups that meet face to face, to virtual communities that share knowledge and information for mutual benefit. You will find information about such groups throughout this book.

Further reading

- Department for Education and Skills (2005) *Getting on in Business, Getting on at Work*. The Stationery Office, London.
- Department of Health (2004) *The NHS Improvement Plan: putting people at the heart of public services*. The Stationery Office, London.
- Department of Health (2004) *Choosing Health: making healthier choices easier*. The Stationery Office, London.
- Department of Health (2004) *National Standards, Local Action: Health and Social Care Standards and Planning Framework 2005/06–2007/08*. www.dh.gov.uk/publications.

Chapter 2

Learning as acquisition

As with most things, ideas about learning vary across time and from place to place, and as with everything else, there is an element of fashion about the multiplicity of approaches. For example, the idea that all (and I mean everyone!) would learn continuously 'from the cradle to the grave' would have horrified our grandparents, who were brought up to expect that post-school learning would be confined to the few, and that even those hardy souls would not require any formal input after the age of about 21.

Ideas about 'lifelong learning' started to emerge in the 1960s in response to perceived inadequacies in existing educational provision. In the 1970s, questions started to be asked by government and business leaders about what learning is *for*. Is it meant to make us better *people* or better *workers*? Since then it feels as if the battle has been won by those who advocate learning for earning – no longer do we learn for the joy and benefit of knowledge for its own sake. Latin has followed Greek in no longer being taught in schools, degree courses are increasingly focused on equipping graduates to find a job, and we are all required to spend our free time enhancing our employability by continually improving our skills.

What kind of learning is this and how does it impact on healthcare workers? If work-related learning is the kind of most concern to the NHS, then some theories about learning are more helpful than others in promoting our understanding of how we can be supportive.

Making sense of the context for work and learning

In this chapter and the next one I would like to introduce some ideas designed to illuminate the various ways in which people learn *for, at* and *through* work, and the likely outcomes in terms of their performance. Before I do this, however, I would like to spend a few moments thinking about where learning happens, because this is crucial to my argument about the importance of good support for learning. Learning *for work* is intended to be preparatory or complementary to the work role, and so it takes place, for example, on initial training courses (pre-registration programmes, apprenticeship courses, etc.). Learning *at work* requires that work be set aside in favour of activities that stimulate or simulate (but do not replicate) work tasks. This can happen in a training room or in front of a PC – the learner is on work premises but is not actually performing the work tasks. Learning *through work* is an integral part of actually doing the job, either individually or within teams or other collective groupings. What will be learned and how it will be applied will differ in each case.

There are many different theories about learning, so it makes sense to focus on those that relate to working. I have organised the most relevant theories into four clusters, and I will indicate where and how these approaches to learning might be identified for use in the workplace. Theories of learning that are relevant to learning *for*, *at* and *through* work can be clustered into four groups as follows:

- learning as behaviour
- learning as understanding
- learning as knowledge construction
- learning as social practice.

This chapter looks at the first two groups, which are broadly concerned with transmitting knowledge and understanding from an expert to a learner. The next chapter takes a different approach, and considers learning as a personal experience that might be facilitated and supported by others in a participatory way, but does not depend on intervention by experts. I shall explore the practical setting of each cluster and the key dilemmas and shortfalls of each cluster as an explanation of learning.

Although all of these broad approaches can be seen in practice, it is worth pointing out that the focus of our interest in this book is the community of learners found in workplaces and generally contained within the social practice cluster (which we cover in Chapter 3). I believe that social theories of learning best describe the kind of learning that will enhance performance and lead to health improvement, although all approaches to learning have a role to play.

Learning as behaviour

This cluster of theories came to prominence in the 1950s, and is associated primarily with the work of BF Skinner, who was a biologist. Skinner argued that a change in behaviour (i.e. learning) is the result of an individual's response to a stimulus, such as being given a piece of information or having a skill demonstrated. A response, such as trying to reproduce the information or copy the skill, will be met with a reward (i.e. praise). A change in behaviour, such as being able to perform the skill, is a demonstration that learning has occurred.

Reinforcement is the key feature of the behavioural theories, and is defined as anything that strengthens the desired response. It could be verbal praise, or a good test result, or a feeling of increased accomplishment or satisfaction.

The behavioural approach has been widely used in clinical settings (for modification of patient behaviour) and in schools (for classroom management), as well as in adult education. The approach is not concerned with transmitting knowledge or with thinking about personal experience, nor is it concerned with the search for meaning and identity on the part of the learner. It is concerned solely with the primed and objective repetition of behaviours.

Let us think about the implications of reinforcement theory in the area of skills development. Practice takes the form of question (stimulus) and answer (response) that exposes the learner to the topic in gradual steps. The learner is conditioned to make a response each time and receives immediate feedback. Learning is ordered in stages of difficulty so that the response to each step is likely to be correct, thus offering opportunities for positive reinforcement. Progress is achieved in small incremental steps which build up towards a positive outcome.

Does this sound familiar? This is how skills have been taught for generations. The learner is introduced to a simple, small task, and is encouraged to master this before moving on to a more complicated task. With expert guidance and feedback, confidence and competence are gained.

Since the 1950s, behavioural theorists have been excited by the possibilities of programmed instruction – in other words, the transmission of content in an orderly, thoughtful sequence using a machine. This has led to the use of technology and the development of modern computer-based training (CBT), which has itself now been eclipsed by Web-based training.

Application of behavioural approaches to learning

The following table gives some examples of contexts in which you will find behavioural approaches to learning, using the idea of learning *for*, *at* and *through* work that I introduced earlier. Expert guidance and bite-sized chunks of learning feature here.

Behaviour	For work	At work	Through work
Approach	Priming	Training	Guiding
Examples	Vocational courses and professional updates	Coaching	Formal direction and feedback
	Short courses, seminars and conferences	Training courses and master classes	Supported practice
		Induction programmes	
		CBT and Web-based training	

Many of the training courses offered to staff working in the NHS are concerned with skills enhancement, and are founded on a behavioural approach to learning. The role of the trainer is that of transmitter of his or her relevant expertise. This approach means that learning outcomes can be written that are specific and measurable and so can be used to support the gathering of evidence of competence. The approach lends itself to e-enabled learning and is prominent in much of the content that has been developed for online delivery. Behavioural approaches can be time – and financially – efficient to deliver and can be adapted to suit the pressures of busy workplaces. It is therefore not surprising that the approach has found favour among trainers. However, there are limits to what can be achieved using behavioural models.

Key dilemmas of this approach

There is no doubt that reinforcement of good behaviour has an important role in enabling learning. However, because this approach requires input from an 'expert', it is usually located away from the workplace and therefore out of context – often based in a classroom. Does learning this way result in learning that can be applied and adapted directly in the workplace? Again, because it takes place away from the workplace, instruction of this kind tends to be discontinuous or 'lumpy' and to be inserted into busy working lives in a 'just-in-time' manner. Its effects can't be easily disentangled from other learning processes that are going on at the same time, such as social learning via discussion with colleagues (discussed more fully in Chapter 3 on pp. 22–3).

A particular dilemma with programmed instruction such as that used in CBT is that its focus on correct responses to fixed circumstances doesn't assist the transfer of skills from one situation to another, nor does it help with the understanding of total situations. By definition, specific content cannot be relevant to all situations, and content that is matched exactly to one task will probably be short-lived and inflexible, given the way that skills now become so rapidly obsolete. However, if instruction is seen as just one aspect of learning, rather than its sole source, we can use a strategy of blending instruction with other forms of learning processes, which we shall explore later.

A further dilemma emerges when we consider the unequal roles and power relationships of the learner and the expert. The suggestion that there is only ever 'one answer' and that it is either known or not known can act as a brake on creativity and self-expression. Dependency on the expert and downplaying of personal knowledge are possible outcomes of this approach to learning.

Learning as understanding

This group of learning theories emphasises the active involvement of the mind in learning. Responses are regarded not as conditioned reactions to stimuli, as we have seen in the behavioural group of theories, but as thoughtful outcomes of perceptions, beliefs and understanding. In contrast to the first group of theories, these theories are about understanding the world rather than just reproducing it, and responding to it appropriately through a process of internalising its principles, concepts and facts. Vastly more complex mental activity is assumed than stimulus–response frames, resulting in the construction, reconstruction and, as necessary, deconstruction of mental models held in the brain.

These theories regard the learner as a powerful information-processing machine whose task is to internalise knowledge about the world. Many theorists have attempted to highlight the key stages of development needed to fulfil this task, in an effort to understand how the brain makes sense and order of so much that is going on around the individual. In the 1980s, with the development of magnetic resonance imaging (MRI) scanners, researchers were able to accumulate a mass of data about how the brain processes information. These data were used by psychologists to develop brain-related approaches to learning. From this has emerged interest in learning styles and the idea that humans possess 'multiple intelligences'. Although there is debate about the usefulness of these concepts, it is clear that brain activity is central to learning.

In order to make sense of the world, development of awareness and understanding can be aided by the processes of facilitation and support, whereby the novice is helped to acquire understanding through appropriate exposure to learning materials, and to solve given problems through guided search. Good facilitation can speed the novice through the developmental stages necessary to achieve mastery of the topic concerned. Since levels of individual understanding will vary significantly from person to person, the facilitator needs to be aware of these differences and to proceed carefully from an acceptable starting point.

Large bodies of knowledge can be made easier to understand by dividing them into an ordered set of blocks (called the curriculum), through which the learner proceeds under their own direction in self-study models, or with the help of a facilitator. CBT and Web-based training offer scope for extensive learner control over pace and style, providing the learner with options with regard to how and what they learn at every point. However, the assumption remains the same – that the body of knowledge presented is 'out there' and must be internalised by the learner so that they can reach the next developmental stage, and in this respect this group of theories differs from the behavioural approach that we examined earlier.

Application of brain-related approaches to learning

This group of theories emphasises the significance of what is 'out there' – that is, the facts and figures that are generally agreed to represent knowledge. The table below shows a few of the ways in which such knowledge and understanding can be gained *for*, *at* and *through* work.

Understanding	For work	At work	Through work
Approach	Engaging	Enriching	Problem solving
Examples	Books, journals and magazines	Case studies, lessons learned and exemplar projects	Analytical frameworks
	Videos, CD-ROMs and multimedia content, Web links	Manuals, codes of practice and internal reports	Knowledge bases
		Benchmarking	Performance support

Learning opportunities that are focused on the acquisition of a body of knowledge, such as that required to enter a profession, will predominantly favour an approach to learning such as I have described here. This kind of knowledge is that which is established and agreed by specialists and experts to be correct. The role of the facilitator becomes that of guide and assistant to understanding, rather than that of offering instruction as previously described. Established knowledge of this kind can be used to write learning outcomes that can be assessed objectively, and this lends itself to e-enabled delivery, allowing the learner to dictate the pace and location of learning. Thus this kind of learning is very useful. However, again there are limitations to the adoption of an approach to learning that is exclusively about aiding the acquisition of knowledge and understanding.

Key dilemmas

We all know people who are very good at knowing the facts but can't put them into practice, and this is the limitation of approaches to learning that emphasise the internalising of knowledge. Such people may display impressive knowledge of the field and perform well in tests, but then fail to perform competently in the work setting. In other words, their knowledge is biased towards *knowing that* rather than *knowing how*. A work-related learning approach needs to make certain that newly acquired knowledge is grounded in practice in order to ensure the development of competence at the same time. One way of achieving this is to blend interventions based on acquiring the facts with learning that encourages their application.

A related dilemma concerns assessment. If learning is just the memorisation of publicly verifiable knowledge, it is a straightforward matter to assess what an individual has 'learned'. Indeed written exams have this very purpose – to assess memory recall rather than potential performance in real situations. And because of the huge variations that exist between people with regard to their experience, understanding, beliefs, attitudes and opportunities, there is a risk that exams of this kind will only test the extent to which the learner has had access to knowledge, rather than their potential to perform in a job role. So school exams test how good the school is as well as how good the learner is – hence the desire on the part of parents to ensure that their children attend the best school available.

Summary

The idea that workplaces can provide a setting for learning has become commonplace over the last decade, as it is acknowledged that our skills have a short life and that we need to constantly learn in order to cope with the dynamic social and economic environment that we now inhabit. This approach first saw the light of day in the 1960s, with the arrival of ideas about 'lifelong learning'. No longer do we learn merely in order to have the joy and satisfaction of knowledge for its own sake. Rather we need to learn in order to earn, and we are encouraged to look upon work and learning as seamless and necessary. But what kind of learning is useful for enhancing our capacity to improve healthcare?

To help our understanding I have drawn a distinction between learning *for*, *at* and *through* work. A great deal of learning as an adult is *for* work, and there is reasonable agreement on what that means. However, it is learning *at* work and learning *through* work that I want to explore, because they are subtly different from each other and lead to very different outcomes. And I believe that it is here in the workplace, during the working day, that the majority of relevant learning will occur, and where support from managers is crucial.

Many people are increasingly of the view that work and learning are overlapping concepts (i.e. learning involves work, and work involves learning). In this chapter I have introduced two different groups of theory that are commonly used to describe learning, and I have given some examples of their use in learning interventions. In the next chapter I shall introduce two more approaches to learning. These are different in that they place the learner at the centre of learning, rather than the expert as has been the case so far.

If you would like to explore behavioural and/or cognitive theories of learning in more depth, I would suggest the following references.

Further reading

- Bandura A (1986) *Social Foundations of Thought and Action: a social cognitive theory.* Prentice Hall, Englewood Cliffs, NJ.
- Dreyfus HL and Dreyfus SE (1986) *Mind over Machine: the power of human intuition and expertise in the era of the computer.* Basil Blackwell, Oxford.
- Skinner BF (1974) *About Behaviourism.* Jonathan Cape, London.
- Skinner BF (2001) *A Brief Survey of Operant Behaviour;* www.bfskinner.org/operant.asp

Chapter 3

Learning as participation

In Chapter 2 we looked at learning that was mediated by expert intervention, and that predominantly required the learner to stop working in
order to learn. There was a structure to the process, and this was decided in
advance, generally by other people. Consider, for example, the learning
that arises from gathering evidence for an NVQ. What is required (and
what is not) is decided by the assessment authority. The way in which
evidence is presented is decided by others. There is a time limit to the
process – learners register, undertake learning, and then submit their
evidence of that learning to match published criteria. The same is true for a
learner undertaking a training day, or registered on a course at their local
college – what is learned and how is decided by others. This is *formal*
learning, and the outcome of such learning is knowledge or skill that is
publicly acknowledged.

Formal and non-formal learning

However, there is another kind of learning that we all engage in
continuously, and which I would like to call *non-formal* learning. Whenever I put the phone down on an unsatisfactory conversation with the
feeling that I didn't get the result I wanted, and I think about how I can do
better next time, I'm doing some learning. When I surf the Internet to find
information, I'm doing some learning. Indeed, like many people, I'm a
totally self-taught IT user. I've learned on a 'just-in-time' basis, and this
has served me well over the years.

If you ask the majority of people how they learned to do their job,
they'll say things like 'by being thrown in at the deep end' or 'by keeping
an eye out for how other people do it'. This is non-formal learning. What is
learned, and its focus and pace, are decided by the individual him- or
herself. This kind of learning is very relevant to job performance – it is
practical and it is related to the specific workplace in which the learner/
worker is operating. It's very personal and incremental – it builds on the
experience of the individual. But of course we none of us work – or learn –
in isolation. We are surrounded by others and we learn by talking and
listening to our colleagues. The two groups of theories that are the subject
of this chapter are about non-formal learning by individuals as part of a
work group.

Learning as knowledge construction

This cluster of theories focuses on the way that people think, test, investigate for themselves and take charge of their own learning on an everyday basis, such that learning is going on continuously and is not separated from interacting with the world around them. This approach challenges the idea that there is such a thing 'out there' as knowledge, independent of the knower. These theories argue that the only knowledge we have is personal to ourselves (and much of it is buried deep in our subconscious), and that learning doesn't involve understanding the 'true' nature of things, but is a personal construction of meaning out of our own experience. The difference between this and the previous group of theories is clear – knowledge is a personal, subjective issue, not something external, 'out there', waiting to be accessed by the individual. Learning is going on all of the time that we are awake – thinking, sifting, prioritising – building on previous knowledge to create new knowledge for ourselves.

Thus knowledge construction is predominantly concerned with activity – learning occurs on an ongoing basis in interactions between the individual and their environment. The social context is crucial in this view of learning, since individual thinking is shaped by active participation in real situations. Because the approach links learning so closely to personal experience, the act of learning becomes inseparable from the construction of meaning. Constructivists believe that knowledge is only usable by a person or a group of people when it has meaning for them (i.e. when it has arisen from their own experiences). Therefore it is the learner who is placed at the centre of the learning experience, rather than the expert instructor (as in the behavioural approach) or the content (as in the brain-focused approach).

Dialogue is recognised as being one of the main ways in which knowledge is constructed, so opportunities for discussion and debate are seen as critical to the learning process. The approach favours hands-on, self-directed activities that lead to debate, design and discovery.

As with the other theories, there is a general recognition that learning can be enhanced through facilitation, although it is not so vital here, as we are all learning all of the time. The task of the facilitator differs – it is not to advise the learner on how to find creative ways of internalising content, but to inspire the learner to discover knowledge for him- or herself. Carl Rogers, one of the first proponents of these theories, believed that you cannot teach a person directly, but that you can only facilitate their learning. Facilitation involves creating an environment in which people can be stimulated to think and act beyond their current level of competence. Ideally learners should be encouraged to think creatively about what the problem is, as well as to think about possible solutions.

Application of constructivist approaches to learning

This approach to learning is significantly different to the other approaches that we have encountered, not least because it enables us to see how close to the workplace we're moving. Here lies the possibility for learning *through work* – integral to the tasks we perform every day. The table below lists some examples of this kind of learning.

Knowledge construction	For work	At work	Through work
Approach	Reflecting	Enquiring	Immersing
Examples	Personal and professional logs	Being mentored	Special projects
	Records of achievement and portfolios	Brainstorming, knowledge sharing and workshops	Job rotations and secondments
	Supported online learning	Discussions with colleagues, customers and suppliers	

As we advance through the clusters of learning theories, we find that the role of the learner and of the supporter of learning (whether we call this person a tutor, a facilitator or a line manager) changes, and the significance of the site of learning becomes more apparent. If we want to encourage everyone to be innovative, to perform better, and to develop their own role while contributing to improved delivery of services, this approach to learning has a lot to tell us. Of course, the level of control over what is learned and how it is learned becomes less for senior managers and greater for the individual. Learning outcomes become less predictable, and there is a greater necessity for regular and informative feedback to learners. However, the learning that occurs is likely to be of much greater value and relevance to individual performance, and the capacity of learners to be flexible, adaptable and innovative is much enhanced. Blending dialogue-favouring approaches to constructing knowledge with the behavioural and/or brain-focused approaches will lead to a more rounded learning experience.

Key dilemmas

This cluster of theories lays great emphasis on the environment in which learning occurs. The potential for learning is helped or hindered by a huge range of what I call 'fuzzy factors' – the organisation, its people, its speed of change, and the level of support surrounding learners while learning is taking place. The job's functions and the way in which they are organised are also crucial. If the worker is isolated, or doing something repetitive all day and every day, the opportunities to be creative and to think about improving their performance, or to experiment with new ideas, are going to be very limited. All of these factors – physical, psychological and social – will exert an influence on what is learned, and this is something that managers need to think about very carefully.

This approach to learning differs in nature from the others in that here we see that knowledge and understanding are entirely personally constructed and dependent on personal experiences, which will differ greatly from person to person. This does not rule out the importance of 'organised' knowledge such as that which we discussed earlier, nor does it suggest that public knowledge doesn't have a place, but it does suggest that the individual will take this public knowledge and adapt it and adopt it to suit their own understanding of the world. If, as knowledge constructionists believe, all meaning is personal, then no idea can be taken as given without due personal understanding. This means that in every meeting, project or other work-related activity, little consistency of thought can be assumed across the group, especially when it contains people of varying age, gender, culture and background. The pursuit of shared vision under such circumstances can be a lengthy affair. There is also a possibility of misunderstanding or conflict unless this is carefully managed. Under the right circumstances the interplay of perspectives can help to increase learning, making the investment of time worthwhile. However, learning in this way is certainly challenging to manage.

Learning as social practice

Our final cluster of learning theories draws attention to the fact that we live in a social world and this influences our understanding. Social theories of learning locate learning in the process of co-operation. They don't contradict the idea of an individual using their brain, or constructing knowledge in their head, nor do they contradict the fact that behaviour has a part to play in conditioning much human activity, but they argue that learning requires a social setting in which to occur, and to be applied. Indeed, many theorists maintain that learning is not just an outcome of social interaction but is integral and inseparable from all of our activities during all of our waking hours.

Social learning theories have become very popular over the last decade and there are a number of versions of them, with supporting evidence from a range of sources. Many theories have been developed by watching how children perform in social settings and how they learn from each other, especially from those slightly older than themselves. Much of this learning is due to imitative behaviour, and this is culturally dependent.

Other theorists have pointed out the vast amount of learning that goes on in activities such as those we see among 'hot teams' who become so accustomed to working together that language becomes superfluous. This can only be achieved through some kind of learning process. However, we don't all work in hot teams. Yet another approach to learning views it as the normal outcome of socialising as we participate in groups, or as we seek out people with similar interests. Learning happens among participants in any community (hot or cold!), and knowledge is embedded within the group. Newcomers acquire, through participation, a sense of how people act in relation to tasks and towards each other, and in doing so they become members of the community themselves.

The idea that participation in a working environment can lead to learned behaviour was described engagingly by Donald Roy. His article, entitled 'Banana Time', concerned a group of people working in the 'clicking room' of a clothing factory (so called because they were assembling zippers, and the machines they used clicked with every movement) learning to remain sane in the face of repetitive work. An identity emerged among the group which gave meaning to the routine tasks. They formed a community and they learned how to support each other, often by playing silly games to help their learning. In one sense the participants were working for each other rather than for the factory, with positive motivational effects.

Application of social practice approaches to learning

Learning in a social context as part of a community has obvious significance for NHS workplaces. To help us to understand what this kind of learning looks like, the table below gives a few examples.

Social practice	For work	At work	Through work
Approach	Networking	Participating in communities	Teamworking
Examples	Professional bodies	Personal networks	Project teams
	Committees, boards and advisory groups	Communities of practice	Functional teams
	Interest groups and associations	Internal committees and management groups	Multi-disciplinary teams
		Action learning sets	Virtual or distributed teams Multi-organisation teams

Socially situated learning of this kind goes on routinely in NHS and social care environments, but often is not recognised as 'learning' because it is not concerned with public (formal) knowledge. As colleagues exchange information and stories about their everyday experience, opportunities arise to build understanding and develop new knowledge. The role and even the identity of the facilitator of learning shifts – now it is more likely to be the line or supervisory manager who is supporting the learning process. Learning outcomes are very difficult to identify, but are likely to be many and varied. Supervisors have a responsibility to engage in discussion ('formative feedback') with learners, but frequently have neither the time nor the skills necessary to do so. This creates a problem. How can we support managers so that they themselves can support learning?

Communities – whether they are focused on sharing ideas or on making practical improvements – are based on the conviction that we learn from each other. We can see some evidence that this is being encouraged in the NHS, but there is still a lot to be done. We need to make it possible for people to share ideas and learn from each other continually as an everyday part of doing their job, and not just on special occasions.

Key dilemmas

The culture found in an organisation is one factor that determines the degree to which people interact, and the degree to which social learning is possible. Everything that is done in an organisation is underpinned by a constantly shifting undercurrent, and this can be seen in how people behave towards each other, and the extent to which people feel comfortable about admitting their concerns and mistakes. This isn't a static situation, but is constantly moving such that traditions, values, policies, beliefs and attitudes are always changing. This draws on the collective energies of everyone involved, constantly seeking to renew and reinterpret itself. In these circumstances the energy required to keep up is such that the sharing of ideas becomes a luxury.

The extent to which a shared understanding can be reached in such a situation is problematic. In busy workplaces, where people are constantly 'running in order to stand still', the difficulty of communicating effectively among the cut and thrust of everyday activity is huge. Think about the NHS ward, kitchen or department, or the average GP surgery, and imagine the extent to which meaningful interaction – and hence meaningful learning – can occur.

The ability of a person to learn through social practice must also depend on their personal disposition and social skills. We rarely choose the people with whom we work, yet our familiarity with those around us must influence how successfully we interact with them and consequently learn.

Given that there are so many ifs and buts, can socially anchored learning ever amount to more than an ad-hoc set of interactions? If this question assumes that learning should be an orderly, controlled experience, drawing on a defined curriculum and working towards a fixed objective, the answer has to be no. However, as a driver of non-formal learning for health improvement in organisations, the potential of an approach based on communities outstrips that of all other theories.

Summary

I would like to conclude by comparing the theories that we have encountered in Chapter 3, which focus on learning from experience both as an individual and as part of a community, with the theories that we met earlier in Chapter 2. First, I hope that all of the approaches sounded familiar to you and that you could recognise the examples I gave of each approach. The first two clusters are concerned with formal, structured learning, which is commonly used on training courses and in education programmes. They are mainly concerned with enhancing learning that can be recognised by a 'reward', which might be praise or a certificate. Such learning is necessary and useful for people at work. The second two clusters focus on what the individual, as part of a group, learns informally while thinking about how they do their job.

As explanations of learning all of these approaches have strengths and weaknesses, and no one approach is sufficient to explain how people learn. When considering them, it's worth bearing in mind the need to build in fitness for purpose when organising learning. If learning is to improve someone's skills or their knowledge base, the behavioural or brain-focused approach takes precedence. However, if we are concerned with health improvement, which I think is a much broader concept, and which involves everyone working in healthcare, then the constructionists in social practice settings have the edge.

The best results with regard to health improvement are likely to be achieved when learning is linked directly to the job, and opportunities are provided for the immediate application of new capabilities. Put simply, behavioural approaches are probably best suited to developing skills, brain-focused approaches to increasing knowledge, constructivist approaches to enhancing performance, and socially mediated learning to accelerating change. In any particular situation, a blend of all four approaches might result in the best overall result. How this can be achieved is the subject of the next few chapters of this book.

To summarise, the table below shows the way I organise the different processes that support learning, and the likely outcomes of each approach.

Learning theories	For work	At work	Through work	Likely outcomes
Learning as behaviour	Courses/ events	Training	Supported practice	Skills
Learning as understanding	Books/ journals	Manuals	Problem solving	Knowledge
Learning as knowledge construction	Reflecting on performance	Being coached	Special projects/ secondments	Performance
Learning as social practice	Networking with peers	Participating with colleagues	Teamworking	Organisational change

Altering the emphasis of healthcare delivery from supply (the service) to demand (the patient) has offered significant benefits. So too, in education and training, it is possible to shift the attention from the expert to the learner, either individually or as part of a group. The table below summarises the varying focus, process and outcome of each of my clusters. It demonstrates that work-related learning for health improvement will be optimised by concentrating on constructivist and socially-situated approaches to learning; those which result in over-arching changes in performance.

	Focus	Process	Outcome
Behaviour	The expert	Reinforcement	Skills
Understanding	The content	Delivery	Knowledge
Knowledge construction	The learner	Activity	Performance
Social practice	The group	Practice	Organisational change

Further reading

- Engestrom Y and Middleton D (eds) (1996) *Cognition and Communication at Work.* Cambridge University Press, Cambridge.
- Rogers CR (1995) *On Becoming a Person: a therapist's view of psychotherapy.* Houghton Mifflin, Boston, MA.
- Roy D (1959) Banana time: job satisfaction and informal interaction. *Hum Organisation.* **18:** 158–68.
- Wenger E (1998) *Communities of Practice: learning, meaning and identity.* Cambridge University Press, Cambridge.

Chapter 4

Managing workplace learning

Learning takes many forms and occurs all of the time and everywhere. Work provides an ever-changing and challenging environment, and non-formal learning is an integral part of everyday interaction. We just have to cast our minds back to the way that work was organised in the NHS 10 or even five years ago, to recognise that we do things very differently these days. We must have learned something in order to cope with it all. Chapters 2 and 3 introduced four different clusters of theories that explain how people learn in order to do their job. The first two approaches focused on the development of skills and understanding. This was achieved through conditioned responses to external stimuli in the first cluster, or via what goes on in people's heads in the second cluster. The clusters discussed in Chapter 3 differed in that they focused on the interactions and experiences of the individual and the group. These approaches argue that thinking is located within actions that alter a situation and thus enable learning to take place. The social context is crucial because it provides a rich array of situations and opportunities. The emphasis here is on individual performance and organisational change.

Work, learning and managerial responsibility

As there is growing pressure on the NHS and social care services to recruit and retain staff and to keep them equipped with flexible and adaptable skills, closer attention is being given to how this second kind of learning can be supported effectively. The Knowledge and Skills Framework and *Agenda for Change* are currently the most prominent example of how this is being shaped. Interest in socially situated learning has developed as it has become recognised that conventional approaches to training tend to mirror the more narrow behavioural approach and therefore do not always address the significant issues that emerge. For example, backfill (substitution of labour) is a potentially enormous problem that makes it seem overambitious to even consider 'developing' everyone. Changing skills requirements make the costs of releasing staff very high, and training courses that are not immediately transferable into day-to-day practice are an inadequate response to a very real need. Alternatives have to be found. Work-based learning modelled on the social practice approach has some significant advantages in terms of resource use and workplace relevance.

Recognition of the need for efficiency and cost-effectiveness, and a growing understanding of the relevance of learning connected with work, have meant that it has become increasingly common to look to the workplace as an appropriate site for learning. Conventional 'training' is increasingly being complemented by innovative approaches to 'learning', often delivered via new and emerging technologies that seem to offer significant advantages in terms of ease of access.

> Learning that is concerned with performance can occur *for*, *at* and *through* work. Learning *for* work might include initial training, conferences and seminars – occasions that take people away from the workplace in order to learn. However, learning *at* and *through* work is generally the way that people learn and understand procedures, protocols and ideas that are relevant and significant *in order to do their job*.

Much learning is now delivered at work. For example, NVQs have been designed to enable people to demonstrate what they can do and to gain recognition for this. One criticism that has been levelled at NVQs is that they are not very developmental of the individual because they emphasise what can already be done. The learning that goes on here may lead to greater self-confidence, and there may be some broadening of the skills base as learners strive to complete the range of activities required to demonstrate competence, but arguably there is not much learning that will develop *new* skills or enable people to become *lifelong learners*.

Work-based learning covers more than just the delivery of NVQs. As was mentioned earlier, most people, if asked how they learned to do their job, will say 'by being thrown in at the deep end' or something similar. Informal learning of this kind is particularly useful for gaining practical skills and for the application of procedures that are directly related to the specific workplace where activity is located. Often our understanding of how to perform at work is instinctive, and is so deeply buried within our consciousness that we don't even realise we possess it. Like driving a car or reading, we don't have to think about how to do it – we just *know how*.

> The range of learning opportunities is growing, but whatever the approach favoured, it is true to say that the success or otherwise of the experience is largely influenced by the people involved (i.e. the worker/learner, fellow workers/learners and their supervisory manager).

Developing such subconscious understanding of the range of knowledge required these days means being exposed to challenge, and having time to reflect on experience. We need to think about how we can do more than simply transfer learning from the classroom to the workplace, but rather create a new kind of learning altogether. Work-based learning of this kind is based on thinking about continual improvement. It is not just about acquiring knowledge and a set of technical skills, but rather it is a case of continually reviewing and learning from experience *while working*. Such work-based learning is about the creation of knowledge as a shared and collective activity whereby people discuss ideas and share problems and solutions. It requires not only the acquisition of new knowledge but also the acquisition of the ability to *learn how to learn*.

If our starting point is that work provides a basis for learning, this has significant implications for how we manage the worker/learner. We are concerned with outcomes that relate to performance – behaviour – as well as those that relate to knowledge and skill, important as they are. The workplace becomes the setting for learning and everyone present has a role to play. However, the success of this kind of learning rests significantly with one person – the supervisory manager – who sets the tone and manages the unfolding of the workplace as a site for learning.

Qualities of the supportive supervisory manager

What are the qualities that supervisory managers need if they want to create, sustain and support an environment in their workplace that will support individual and group learning?

Workplaces differ, and so do the people who work in them. Supervisory managers approach their role in a variety of ways. Some are very supportive of those for whom they are responsible, seeing them as individuals with varying needs who require differing levels of support in order to do their job and to learn, develop and share their increasing understanding with others. Such a manager is Joe Bloggs, who is not very experienced as a manager, but has a clear vision about what he wants his team to achieve, and is very motivated to create an atmosphere at work that will support a team approach.

Other managers take a very task-oriented approach to their management responsibility. Jane Bell is a manager with long experience of the job and of managing others, but does not have the insight to help her to get the best from her team. How and why are these people different? In this chapter I shall look at some of the qualities that make a manager and see if this helps to differentiate between Joe and Jane. This might help us to identify the elements that contribute to a supportive environment for learning in the workplace, and the role of the supervisory manager in helping or hindering its development.

Watching Joe and Jane at work we could observe the following:

Joe	Jane
• Is good at 'horizon scanning'	• Is good at 'firefighting'
• Keeps abreast of changes in the NHS	• Focuses on throughput, targets and tasks
• Is keen to network whenever possible	• Is too busy to stop and have a chat
• Recognises his own weaknesses	• Has been doing the job for years, and knows that the tried and tested solutions always work
• Watches how other managers manage	• Has been in this job the longest and knows all the wrinkles
• Has a personal career strategy	
• Asks colleagues and team members for feedback on his own performance	• Is confident that her methods are effective
• Involves them in and listens to them during decision making	• Is always keen to get people to 'play the game'
• Helps individual learning linked to skills needed in the workplace	
• Supports team learning	

An accomplished manager is one who is **ready, willing** and **able** to put into **practice** ideas about workplaces as places to learn with the **understanding** required to operate a style of managing to support this. They are:

- **ready** to pursue a vision of the workplace as a community of mutually supportive people
- **willing** to expend the energy and persistence necessary to sustain such a community
- **able** to learn from their own and others' experiences through reflection on actions and their consequences
- **practice** oriented in order to transform their vision, motives and understanding into a functioning reality
- **understanding** of the concepts and principles needed to sustain such an approach.

We can think of the supervisory manager who is concerned with supporting learning as having the qualities shown in Figure 4.1.

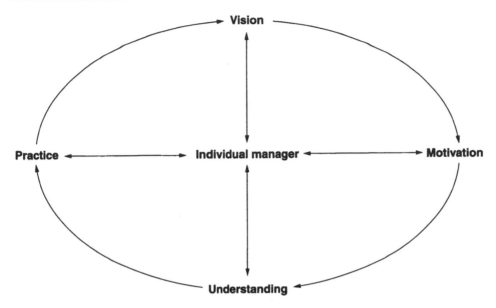

Figure 4.1 Qualities of the supportive manager.

Vision

Having a shared vision among the team is often said to be *the* most important ingredient for delivery of an excellent service, because it breeds shared commitment, and it results in joint actions and effort. Where does this vision come from if not from the supervisory manager who motivates the team and generates and discusses relevant ideas? An appropriate vision – a 'big idea' – provides an ideal that can be shared by everyone in the team and has the capacity to unite people around shared aspirations. This makes vision an important driver of staff performance.

Even if they aren't aware of it, all managers have a set of beliefs about how to manage. Often they have acquired this from the experience of themselves being managed in the past. Supportive managers generally see managing as a process that doesn't involve *telling* people what to do, but one in which discussion enables people to recognise what is needed – to enable learning as a *process*, not just of repeating or restating what is required.

How would we know a visionary manager if we saw one?

Motivation

Supportive managers are able to recognise what motivates staff to learn and to perform effectively, and can build on this to foster further learning, giving people a sense of achievement, recognition and respect. However, it isn't easy, because workplace motivation is a complex issue. Although people need to feel that they are being financially rewarded in an appropriate way, they also need to feel that their contribution to the organisation and its goals is recognised – that their learning, and thus their good performance, will be rewarded by added responsibility, status or promotion, making it worthwhile to invest in their own learning. They need to feel that they can use new capabilities by participating in interesting and novel work activities, and in successful delivery of the service.

A manager can have a vision of good management based on role models, and be unhappy with the majority of managing that they see around them. However, they can be unable to move towards better practice, and unsure of what to do. They can be insufficiently motivated to change, and feel inadequately supported by their workplace or peers to take the risks to be different, or to make the effort to change. We all know how big the gap between wanting to lose weight and actually going on a diet can be!

> What tips the balance that moves a manager from wanting to be supportive to actually demonstrating support?

Understanding

Putting a personal vision into practice and motivating staff to learn requires more than just sending them on training courses. It requires the supervisory manager to understand the difference between propositional knowledge (the facts, regulations and theories needed to perform appropriately) and procedural knowledge (the organisational, socially constructed protocols that make a workplace 'tick') and what is fit for purpose as far as learning is concerned. It requires the supervisory manager to understand how to support learning *at* and *through work*, how to encourage people to share their knowledge with others, and how to inspire people to want to learn more – and contribute more – to the success of the service. Supervisory managers need to be able to give people a sense of purpose by allowing them to organise their learning, and then their improved work capability, for themselves rather than imposing a culture of supervision and training. Consistent and practical support for learning within their workplace will achieve this.

An accomplished manager is not only inspired, enlightened and motivated, but must also be skilled in putting ideas into practice. An accomplished manager will understand what has to be achieved as well as how to achieve it – they must *know* and be able to *do*. They must recognise and utilise their staff's strengths.

What are the paths towards knowing and doing, and can they be trodden?

Practice

An accomplished manager is not only ready, willing and knowledgeable, but is also able to live the vision – to 'walk the talk' – which is enormously complex. This style of managing makes great demands on the performance of managers because it requires the skills of assessing the performance of others, guiding and supporting them towards better performance, and helping them to share their growing understanding with others in the team.

However, the benefit of developing individuals and groups who can take responsibility for their own actions and learning, and who will continue to learn, far outweighs the extra effort required.

How can we motivate managers to put into practice their vision, their knowledge and their skills with regard to supporting the learning of others in the workplace?

Summary

In this chapter we have shifted the focus from the individual learner towards the environment within which they are learning, and we have started to think about the relationship between the line manager and the learner. Health improvement depends on organisational change, and this will only come about by providing circumstances within which effective learning can occur. Whole system change requires the involvement of everyone, and the supervisory manager is pivotal in enabling a holistic approach.

Jane Bell is a good manager and she has been in post for many years. She probably runs an efficient department and has no doubt been praised for this by senior management. She is surrounded by people every day, but she doesn't inhabit a community, and those who report to her are unlikely to feel that they are a team or are making a contribution to health improvement, because they are primarily 'doing the job' with their hands and not with their minds. Joe Bloggs, however, takes a very different approach. He is able to focus on developing solutions that are of strategic importance, because he has developed a relationship of trust and empowerment among his staff and colleagues.

I have outlined the attributes that Joe embodies and that help him in his approach to supporting the learning of others. Joe would probably be surprised to be told that he is supporting learning, because as far as he is concerned he is simply practising good managerial skills. However, his approach is such that his colleagues feel encouraged to be innovative and to talk to each other about uncertainties, including the future direction of the service and their role within it.

Health improvement can only come about if staff are committed to the concept and are enabled to make a contribution by learning, sharing and progressing. In the next chapter a number of 'dilemmas' will be presented that are fairly common problems for the supervisory manager, and a range of responses will be suggested. Will you be a 'Joe' or a 'Jane'?

Further reading

- Argyris C (1994) *On Organisational Learning*. Basil Blackwell, Oxford.
- Schultz TW (1961) Investment in human capital. *Am Econ Rev.* **51**: 1–17.
- Senge PM (1990) *The Fifth Discipline: the art and practice of the learning organisation*. Doubleday, New York.

Chapter 5

Dilemmas

Problems and issues about learning come in many shapes and forms, and are sometimes difficult to recognise. Clues are available, but the way in which they are used varies, and outcomes differ accordingly. This chapter presents a few typical scenarios ('dilemmas') that the supervisory manager might face when trying to support learning. They are offered in the hope that they will provoke reflection and discussion and encourage the development of innovative solutions to common problems. The chapter provides you with an opportunity to test your capacity as a supervisory manager to support learning, against a number of hopefully realistic scenarios. Joe and Jane from the previous chapter would certainly know how to respond in each case, but the likelihood is that they would respond differently. What do you think? And how might your views differ from those of your colleagues?

Dilemma I

In 2001 a note came round from the Director of Resources at the trust which said that all of the lads in my team had to undergo training in risk management. The training consisted of six half-day workshops with some preparatory reading in between, and at the end everyone had to take a test to demonstrate what they knew about the subject they had been learning about. This was a mandatory course, and it was going to be offered twice a year to make sure that new starters had a chance to attend, and to enable those who had failed the first time to have another go. However, it was a case of 'three strikes and you're out'. Anyone who couldn't pass the test after three attempts would lose their job.

One of the lads in my team – Chris Smith – was very loud in condemning all of this 'management stuff', pointing out that we had had no accidents on our shift for the 10 years that he'd worked for the trust, and wasn't that evidence enough that we were all capable of doing our job? I had to point out to him that it wasn't just our team – it was everybody working for the trust – and that there had been plenty of near misses in other areas of the trust. What about that time last year when the gardeners nearly had a very nasty accident with some chemical fertilisers they had been using? Chris wasn't convinced. He's a nice lad – he's always cheerful and very helpful to staff and patients, he always has a smart word and is good at the repartee, and he can always tell you which team's likely to win the league and which manager is going to get the sack soon! He's always taken an interest in politics and is very active in the Union. I've always felt that he could go far with a bit of application, but I'm pleased that he hasn't because he's been very useful to me over the years.

I was very surprised on the first day of the course when Chris turned up late, sat at the back and didn't murmur a word during the opening session. In fact he was so quiet that I didn't notice that he wasn't there after coffee until one of the other lads pointed it out. Chris missed the second and third workshops because he had problems at home (most unlike him, as he was very rarely late or off work). He turned up very late for the test – saying that he had overslept – and was not allowed to take it. So he had to wait until the next round four months later. The pattern then was even worse. He just went missing during the workshops and didn't turn up for the test either. Nothing I said or did seemed to make any difference – there was always an excuse.

So we are just about to start on his third attempt. If he fails this time he'll lose his job, and that would be a disaster for Chris and his wife and kids.

What should I do?

- Pretend I haven't noticed that he's in danger of losing his job and say nothing?
- Start disciplinary proceedings because of his poor attendance at previous courses, in the hope that this will shock him into attending this time?
- Offer to bring forward his promised promotion to team leader if he is successful with the course?
- Or what do you suggest?

What will be the likely outcome of each choice?

Dilemma 2

I don't know why it is, but there's always something happening at the surgery – something that keeps the stress levels high, no matter how hard we try to anticipate the unexpected.

Take that incident last month when Jo Brown was nearly attacked by the son of one of our patients. That was a very nasty thing to happen to anyone, and Jo is so thoughtful about her patients – she's the last person you'd want to see harmed. She's been a district nurse for a long time (probably about 20 years), and she'll always go out of her way to help. On this occasion it was late and she'd been on the go all day and well into the evening when the call came that Mrs X wanted to see her urgently. Jo didn't give it a second thought, and rushed straight round to be confronted by Mrs X's son, who hadn't taken his medication and was just about off his head. He took exception to the look of Jo – probably the uniform – and lashed out. Poor Jo had a nasty set of bruises but it could have been much worse.

Then there was the time when Jill, our physiotherapist, became so very entangled in the needs of her patients that she nearly had a breakdown herself. It came to a head when she had to visit that nice journalist woman who was in remission with breast cancer, but who was going downhill again. Poor Jill had spent an inordinate amount of time with this patient when she needed remedial exercise, and she'd become very close to her, although she knew that this was a little unprofessional. However, the patient was living on her own, and was similar to Jill in age and circumstances, and I suppose Jill had spent such a lot of time in her company that it was inevitable that they should share confidences. When Jill heard that the patient had collapsed and been rushed into hospital she was distraught.

Sometimes, of course, the stress gets to us and we take it out on each other. Accommodation at the surgery isn't very good. It's an old Victorian house that was converted years ago – it looks pretty from the outside but is very cramped and run down inside. Many of our staff are attached to several surgeries in the primary care trust, so they might only spend one session per week here, and they have to share offices and consulting rooms. This shouldn't be so bad, but they all have different standards of tidiness, and they rarely see each other. In fact we often find that they are visiting the same people but are unaware of this. The family that gave Jo Brown such a fright had been visited the day before by a health visitor who had come to see the newest member of the family. She had been threatened by Mrs X's son (who was the father of the child), but of course it hadn't occurred to her to mention this, as she rushed from place to place.

As the practice trainer I can see that we'd all be less stressed if we worked together as a team rather than as ships that pass in the night. But what can I do?

- Use some of my tight budget to organise an away-day with an expert facilitator who will train everybody in communication skills?
- Lobby for a bigger building that can accommodate us all?
- Spend money on an email system so that we can keep in touch with each other?
- Or what do you suggest?

How can I support shared learning when the team doesn't even meet?

Dilemma 3

I've been in post for just over a year now, and I feel that I've achieved quite a lot, but I must confess that some things still defeat me. For example, take the problem I'm having with Marie, which could undo all of the effort I've put into improving service over the last year.

Like many others, Accident and Emergency struggles to meet targets on waiting times, and I came into post with plenty of ideas about how this situation could be changed. For example, I'm aware of some work that was done in the North-East in response to the NHS Performance Assessment Framework that was published in 1999. They focused on efforts to shorten admission times for elderly people with fractured neck of femur. They looked at the patient journey and found that time was wasted as patients waited for porters to transport them to the X-ray department, then bring them back, then transport them to the ward for admission, and so on. They found that by giving responsibility to a nurse to assess and then accompany the patient throughout their journey, and by allocating a porter to remain with the patient from arrival to admission, and by allowing the radiographer to make a diagnosis, they were able to reduce the number of repeat journeys to and from Accident and Emergency and shorten waiting times. Their results were astounding – from an average of 4% meeting their target of admission within an hour, they achieved a rate of about 70% almost overnight.

I thought that this was something we could easily do. I worked hard to persuade the powers that be to fund the development of a training course that would prepare staff for these changes. I commissioned this from the university, and I have to say that they did a brilliant job. There was none of this old-fashioned training in the classroom stuff. Instead they came up with an amazing online programme, very whizzy with lots of information, links to some brilliant sites, graphics, self-tests – you name it, it was there. The course could be accessed by staff anywhere, at any time, and only took 10 hours to complete. I thought it would solve all of our problems.

Then Marie said that she didn't think it was a good idea, and she spread all manner of gossip about it being designed to reduce the number of staff and to get more out of those who remained, getting people to do what they weren't qualified to do, and so on. However, she didn't say this to me – instead she talked to everyone else at every opportunity. Consequently there was a lot of uncertainty and there was a very dark atmosphere around the coffee room.

So I spent time talking to everyone in turn, explaining the reason for the changes, and asking them to work through the programme, in their own time, but by the end of March. There were grumbles – some people went away prepared to give it a go, but quite a few were clearly unconvinced and the grumbles were still heard. And Marie? She said that she didn't have time for this kind of stuff, as she had a family to care for (that's why she worked nights, so that she could look after the kids during the day). She didn't have a computer at home, and she wasn't prepared to go to the Learning Resource Centre during her shift, as it was at the back of the hospital grounds, and pitch dark and silent (I don't blame her – I'd be nervous, too).

What can I do?

- Forget the whole thing?
- Arrange a transfer for Marie?
- Talk to the Human Resource (HR) department about having her disciplined for insubordination?
- Or what do you suggest?

How can I introduce changes when people and systems can't or won't change?

Dilemma 4

It seems hard to believe, but some of my staff are *too* keen! What do you do when everyone takes the message about lifelong learning very seriously, and all of them want to develop themselves, and do it *now*?

I am the departmental manager of the radiography department here. We're a middle-sized department with a friendly atmosphere, and we all work well together. The trust is fortunate in being able to train and retain staff with better than average success. People tend to stay around here and generally have well-established roots – it's a fairly quiet part of the country and there's still a strong feeling of community. I guess it stems from the time when we had a lot of heavy industry and men worked shifts while their wives stayed at home to look after the family. Of course things have changed a lot since the coalmines and the shipyards were closed down. These days it's as likely as not that the wives are the breadwinners and the men are house-husbands. Women have taken up the challenge and really enjoy the freedom to work and better themselves (I'm not sure what the husbands think!).

In a sense that's the underlying problem for me. I have some really good staff and I want them to feel that I'm supporting them, but resources are limited and it's hard to avoid disappointing some of them. Before 2002 it wasn't my concern, as all training budgets were held centrally and most of the resources went to a few professional groups – medics and nurses tended to do well, whereas paramedics and support staff seriously missed out. Either there weren't enough of them to give them any clout, or they weren't really interested in training. For example, Individual Learning Accounts (ILAs) were on offer for a long time but there was very little take-up.

The HR department was reorganised in 2002 when a new director of HR was appointed. He was keen that the trust should be seen to be inclusive, and he was particularly enthusiastic about encouraging lifelong learning. He decided that training budgets would be devolved to individual departmental level, and that departmental managers would have discretion about how the budget was spent. We were all very pleased with this turn of events, because we could see that it would help us to plan our skills mix and ensure that succession planning could be improved.

It has worked very well on the whole, but there have been some issues, and my present problem has been rumbling for some time. Now it has come to a head. It is partly a consequence of the very limited career structure in radiography. Once staff have qualified, they have only a few opportunities for upgrades and extra responsibility. If they want to keep developing themselves as professionals they can diversify by training in the use of other media (ultrasound, nuclear magnetic resonance scanning, CAT scanning, etc.), but this can only be done by registering on recognised training courses, which are expensive. Many people who are really keen do Masters courses, but then they find that these don't give them any advantage in terms of career unless they move jobs. There is still a tendency to appoint the longest-serving member of staff to senior vacancies, all other things being equal.

Which brings me to Ann and Cathy. They've been friends for years – both trained here and stayed, got married, had families and came back to work. Both are loyal and caring members of staff, and both are ambitious. They both feel that the time is right to embark on Masters degree programmes. Ann wants to do a management course and Cathy wants to do a course that will broaden her professional skills. Both can do such courses through the local university, part-time over two years, with minimum disruption to their family life, and it suits both families for them to start soon. However, budgets are finite. I can't send both of them on the funds I have available. There is the slim possibility that if I make a case to the HR department there may be some discretionary finance at the end of the financial year. However, if I do this it means that no other member of staff in my department, and possibly deserving others in other departments, will be able to do any training for the next two years.

What should I do?

- Tie up budgets for the foreseeable future in recognition of both staff members' loyalty?
- Insist that only one of them can do a Masters degree for the next two years, and that they must sort out who that is between themselves?
- Send neither of them and use the budget to allow all staff to receive some training over the next two years?

- Or what do you suggest?

What might be the consequences of my actions?

Dilemma 5

I am a big believer in helping others, and I think that, since we spend such a large proportion of our lives at work, we should do everything we can to make it as pleasant as possible. This philosophy has stood me in very good stead over the years, and although I'm not particularly well qualified, I've worked my way up so that I'm now in quite a senior position in the admissions department of the hospital. Some people think it's rather boring, but I always find something to keep my interest alive and I've met some really nice people over the years. It's very busy of course, and you have to keep on top of all of the rules and regulations – it can be stressful and it doesn't suit everyone. We have a high rate of staff turnover, so there's always someone new to get to know.

I suppose I have a reputation as a 'people person', and that's fine. My home life is a little on the quiet side, and work is where I do my socialising, so naturally when new people start I do all that I can to help them to settle in. The HR department asked me to join in a new venture they wanted to set up last year, namely a mentoring scheme. They said that they were only choosing people who would be good mentors, and that they would give them some training so that they would know what to do. It sounded pretty much what I'd been doing anyway, so I was more than happy to let my name go forward.

They gave us the training, which lasted for two days, and there was a file of reading to go with it. Unfortunately I didn't have time to go through it very carefully, but I got the general idea of what was wanted. They allocated me someone to mentor, and they suggested that we should both meet up for coffee and get to know each other. After that it was up to us how often we met and what we talked about.

Everything went well at first. The woman they gave me to mentor – Frances – was very pleasant. She is about my age and has been working here for about nine months. She works in one of the clinics and I'm very friendly with her manager, Doris (we've known each other for years). It was nice to know that there was a reason to have coffee together, and we agreed to meet soon after the scheme started. Frances clearly got a lot from the conversation, because she suggested that we meet again the next day for lunch. In fact I was busy that day, but we sorted something out and I thought things were set fair.

When I mentioned Frances to Doris she groaned and said that Frances was a hopeless case – totally disorganised and with no attention span at all. Anything I could do for her would be welcomed, not just by Doris but by all the other long-suffering people who had to work with her. I soon learned that Frances was totally unreliable, and she often failed to turn up for meetings we'd arranged. At other times she would just pop in unannounced and expect me to stop whatever I was doing to talk to her. She was very grateful for all of the advice I gave her, and after a couple of months Doris remarked that Frances' performance was improving. I was really pleased that I was able to do something to help.

After a while Frances and I got into a rhythm of meeting, and she shared more and more of her problems with me. She always listened carefully to my advice, and she said that she did what I suggested and it usually worked. After a time we started to meet after work for a bite to eat, and a couple of times we went to the cinema. Her home life was very turbulent. She started to tell me things that I really didn't want to know about herself and her husband, who sounded like a real terror, and her children, who were rather wild. Some of the things she was telling me were shading into criminality. I told her what I thought in no uncertain terms – that she should sort things out at home in order so that she would be able to concentrate on her job, even if it meant leaving her husband.

It seems that she told him what I had been saying, because she's just popped across from the clinic to tell me that he's waiting outside to 'sort me out'.

What should I do?

- Go out and confront him?
- Call the police?
- Sneak out of the back door and resign from the mentoring scheme?
- Or what do you suggest?

What did I do wrong and how can I improve?

Dilemma 6

I am the divisional manager for Estates and Facilities for three acute hospitals that make up one large trust. One site is a large district general hospital, and there are two smaller, older, local sites. I am responsible for organising the work of Estates staff, which includes all ancillary workers, such as porters, domestic staff, chefs, ward hostesses and Health Care Assistants (HCAs). The numbers vary as we are constantly being restructured, and we always have a big list of vacancies, but generally there are about 400 people for whom I am responsible.

Like most trusts these days we have real issues with recruitment and retention. Gone are the days when we could rely on a regular supply of housewives (and then their daughters) to work shifts as cleaners and cooks. We are now in competition with the big superstores and sandwich factories for staff, and they offer paid holidays and good training to everyone. In days gone by we used to have people who were proud to work for the hospital, which they thought of as 'theirs', and who were pleased to come to work, do a good job and then go home again. If the job was a bit messy or repetitive, that was just to be expected. It was regular work, and they all felt part of a close-knit community. But then sub-contracting was introduced, which meant squeezes on pay and loss of benefits such as paid leave, and this has had real knock-on effects over the years.

The jobs in Estates have changed. They used to be of the kind that you could more or less walk in from the street and set to work straight away, whereas now the machines and the rules and regulations are such that you sometimes almost need to be an Einstein to cope with them all. And over the last couple of years we've had scares such as MRSA and the like which have made everyone look more closely at what goes on in this part of the service. Not surprisingly, they found that staff here are generally getting on a bit – very few younger people are satisfied with the idea of a job in a laundry – so there's going to be trouble ahead as increasing numbers retire and there is no one to take their place. Estates staff have never had much in the way of training or support, and as the conditions for other staff groups have improved, we have been left more and more behind.

The trust decided that something should be done. They commissioned a review and, I have to admit, they listened carefully to what was said by everyone involved. The recommendation was that everyone working in the trust, including those in Estates, should have access to good training backed up by annual appraisals and personal development plans (PDPs). To get over issues such as backfill and costs, e-learning was presented as the solution, but it had to be carefully positioned so that it was genuinely for everyone. The trust invested heavily in setting up an e-learning facility. They bought 10 PCs and they set up an open-plan area next to the canteen so that everyone who ate their meals on site walked past and saw what was available. They bought a huge range of training packages and they employed one woman full-time to act as manager and trainer to help anyone who wanted help with the technology.

At first some interest was shown by staff, but before long this petered out and now, whenever you walk past, the place is deserted, with only the training manager sitting there surfing the Internet. I've asked people why they don't use the computers and they say things like 'the woman is always hovering ready to pounce', 'mates will think I'm getting above myself if they see me there', 'the courses don't suit my needs' and 'they're all to benefit the trust – such as Health and Safety – what do I want with that?'.

It worries me that the trust will see this as a waste of money and will be even more reluctant to invest in training next time.

What should I do?

- Put pressure on all staff to sign up for a course?
- Work with the trainer to produce some marketing material?
- Find a small group of enthusiasts and encourage them to start things off?
- Get my fellow managers to sign up with me for a course to set an example?
- Or what do you suggest?

What will be the likely consequences of each of my actions?

Summary

There are any number of situations that the committed supervisory manager confronts and resolves on a daily basis. Occasionally the solution is an obvious one, so the sticky issues can be tackled and resolved, allowing everyone to move on. Frequently, however, there is no one 'right' answer, but only a number of alternative solutions. Whichever of these is chosen will have consequences both for the people and for the organisation involved.

Most managers find their own ways of dealing with such dilemmas that arise regularly at work. This chapter presents a few common problems that managers encounter where the solution is not an obvious one. Thinking ahead about all of the possible routes to resolution and sharing ideas with others can lighten the burden. Recognising that workplace learning brings its own bundle of dilemmas, but that there are ways of handling them effectively, can help the supervisory manager to support learning to maximum effect.

Further reading

- Argyris C (1976) *Increasing Leadership Effectiveness*. John Wiley & Sons, New York.
- Dennison WF and Kirk R (1990) *Do, Review, Learn, Apply: a simple guide to experimental learning*. Basil Blackwell, Oxford.
- Dobbs K (2000) Simple moments of learning. *Training*. 37: 52–4.

Chapter 6

The significance of the workplace

How supportive of learning are you?

You may never have thought about your own skill in supporting learning, so here is an opportunity to test yourself. Answer the questions below by rating yourself on a scale of 1 to 4 as follows:

This applies to me:

– to a considerable extent	1
– to a moderate extent	2
– to a slight extent	3
– not at all	4

Vision

Having a clear vision of what makes a workplace supportive of learning will enable me to support learners, because I will be able to create a shared direction of travel.

- My operational plans are informed by a specific model of the likely skills mix that will be required of my team in the next two to three years.

1	2	3	4

- I think about incidents and people at work during my off-duty time, and this often results in new ideas about how to approach my job.

1	2	3	4

- I spend time helping members of my team to develop a worked-up plan of where and how they will progress their career development.

1	2	3	4

- In the past I have changed the way in which I organise work with my team as a result of something I have read or discussed with colleagues.

1	2	3	4

If you want to know more about the vision required of a supervisory manager, *see* p. 31.

Motivation

Supportive managers know what motivates staff to learn, and can build on this to foster further learning.

- I am surrounded by people who seem fulfilled by, proud of and committed to their job, and who enjoy working with other people on shared challenges.

1	2	3	4

- Members of my team demonstrate a sense of ownership over their work and have the confidence to act on their own initiative.

1	2	3	4

- I find that I can predict the outcome of incidents related to work and people, and I know how these incidents can be managed.

1	2	3	4

- I believe that the day-to-day work and success of people in my team has a positive impact on patient outcomes.

1	2	3	4

If you want to know more about the motivation of supervisory managers and staff, *see* p. 32.

Understanding

A supportive supervisory manager understands how to tap into the motivation of others to encourage them to share their learning with others.

- I am frequently surprised by the breadth of skills that people display.

| 1 | 2 | 3 | 4 |

- I believe that people themselves create an atmosphere at work that makes it easy to share their knowledge.

| 1 | 2 | 3 | 4 |

- People come to me with ideas that they think would improve work productivity and/or outcomes.

| 1 | 2 | 3 | 4 |

- I am occasionally aware of unexpressed issues at work that I can influence and change.

| 1 | 2 | 3 | 4 |

If you want to know more about the understanding required of supervisory managers, *see* p. 32.

Practice

An accomplished manager is not only ready, willing and knowledgeable, but is also able to live the vision – to 'walk the talk'.

- I encourage team members to develop new learning opportunities and to apply what they have learned.

| 1 | 2 | 3 | 4 |

- I go out of my way to demonstrate interest in the progress of people who are registered on development programmes at work.

1	2	3	4

- I talk to my manager colleagues about issues to do with supporting those individuals for whom I am responsible.

1	2	3	4

- I take my own professional development seriously.

1	2	3	4

If you want to know more about how you can practise the skills of supporting learning as a supervisory manager, *see* p. 33.

Test scores and what they mean

The above self-test was divided into four categories:

- vision
- motivation
- understanding
- practice.

Let's review your score.

If on the test you scored mostly 1s in the first section, this suggests that you have a clear *vision* of the future relating to work and where you wish to take your team. You are aware of the current strengths among staff for whom you are responsible, and you recognise that forward planning will ensure that you retain complementary and appropriate skills among your team. You are flexible and adaptable in your thinking and planning, and ready to respond to the unexpected changes that will inevitably occur in healthcare settings.

If you scored mostly 1s in the second section, this suggests that you are *motivated* to provide a supportive environment for learning, and that you are sensitive to what motivates others. This results in a workplace where staff feel fulfilled and committed to both their job and their workmates, and where they feel empowered to take control of their own activity.

If you scored mostly 1s in the third section, this suggests that you have a deep *understanding* of the needs of learners. A manager with such understanding would know how to build on the motivation and commitment of learners to encourage them to share their ideas so that others will benefit. Understanding of people and of workplace cultures is necessary if supervisory managers are to truly encourage learning through work.

If you scored mostly 1s in the fourth section, this suggests that you not only know how to motivate and support others, but that you are able to put your knowledge and skill into *practice*, for the benefit of those learners for whom you are responsible. It also suggests that you are aware of your own needs both as a manager and as a learner.

You may have found that in some categories you scored 2 or 3 more often than 1. This might be so for a number of reasons. The supervision of others might be a new responsibility for you, or you may be working under such pressure that you don't have time to think about the bigger picture and where your staff fit within it. Maybe you have been doing your job for a long time, so your approaches have become routine. Whatever the reason, the fact that you have read this far in the book is a positive step, and should help you to think more creatively about how you support learning in future.

To enable you to find out more about the ideas behind this quiz, I would like to invite you to read and reflect on the ideas contained in these pages. You may wish to return to the 'dilemmas' in Chapter 5 and review your responses to the scenarios in the light of your capacity to articulate a vision and to motivate others, your understanding of the issues and the opportunities you have to put these ideas into practice. The ideas that I write about here are not intended to give you the 'right' answers, because the management of others is never clear-cut. Supportive management of learning requires creativity and responsiveness. Rather, this book is designed to raise your awareness of some of the issues, and to encourage you to learn more about the vital role that you are fulfilling as a supportive supervisory manager.

The workplace as a site for learning

Over and above vision, motivation and understanding, a supportive manager needs to be able to reflect on and learn from experience in order to put into practice a desire to support the learning of others. First, they must become more aware of their own disposition and performance. The accomplished manager is one who smoothly integrates vision, motivation, understanding and practice into the enactment of managing, and who learns to improve continually through active reflection. Managing requires thoughtful, reflective and purposeful action.

However, managers are not acting in a vacuum. They inhabit an environment at work that either helps or hinders their own development as supportive and community-oriented managers. People shape their organisations, and those organisations in turn shape them. All managers build on their previous experience and are influenced by what is going on around them.

> To what extent do individual managers in your organisation learn to use a management style that conforms with the practices that they see around them?

To represent the interaction of the individual manager and the community of managers, we need to add an additional layer to our model of management for health improvement which I introduced on p. 29. Figure 6.1 puts the manager, along with his or her values, in the environment within which everyday actions are played out. We can see that individual vision, motivation, understanding and practice sit within a workplace community where a variety of visions, motivations, practices and commitments are to be found. There may be a sense of shared endeavour, or there may be differences that can impact on how learning is supported. Exploring these topics as part of a community of supervisory managers can result in greater understanding and strengthened support for everyone.

> How much harmony is there between the individual and the group of managers in your organisation? How does that affect the way in which the individual manager performs his or her management role?

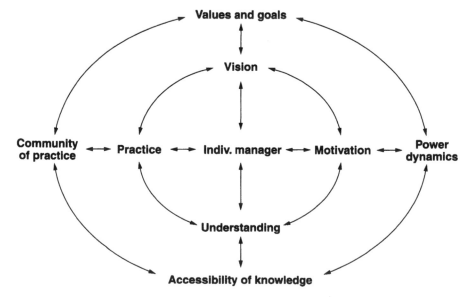

Figure 6.1 Interface of the individual supervisory manager and the community of managers.

Values and goals

At the beginning of this book we talked about the *NHS Improvement Plan* and its focus on patient choice, a theme that runs throughout the book. This is an example of an overarching organisational goal that can only be successfully achieved if the 'big idea' is reflected in the day-to-day reality of the everyday workplace in the NHS. Every employee of the NHS, if asked, would agree that patients and end users of the service are important and that they should dictate both how the service is run and what its purpose should be. However, the translation of policies into actions is often fraught with difficulty, partly because the outcome depends on interpretation by a series of managers before it arrives at the point of action – the patient–service interface. There are always contrary pressures, tensions and priorities involved. It can seem like Chinese whispers when closely examined – intentions get skewed and outcomes can be surprising. Thus achieving a situation in which values and goals are agreed and put into action is not straightforward. The values and goals of the individual supervisory manager may not coincide with those of the community of supervisory managers, or with those who make the overarching decisions that affect how the service is run. This can add further complexity to the role of supervising the learning of others.

> Can you think of an example of a situation where you found yourself in conflict with others in your organisation, particularly in relation to your personal values or goals?

Power dynamics

We have discussed a number of motivating factors that influence individual learners, and the way in which supervisory managers can use ideas about motivation to support learning. At the same time we have recognised that supervisory managers are themselves learners and also require support. Equally, we have to recognise that workplaces are contested environments – factors such as status, age, gender and personality all influence who is listened to and whose ideas are enacted. How all of this is played out in the workplace will affect what is learned and what is applied and shared. However, we should not automatically assume that the dynamic is always negative. If there is openness and transparency, shared values, and commitment to an ideal of lifelong learning for all, power can be benignly exercised. Supervisory managers are influential, and they play an important part in establishing an organisational dynamic. Acknowledging this and developing strategies to build on the power structures that exist can be helpful in fostering an environment within which learning is supported. A group of managers working together towards this ideal will achieve more than any individual manager could.

> The idea of a 'benign use of power' is an interesting one. Have you had any experience of this?

Accessibility of knowledge

In order to offer appropriate support for learning in the workplace, the supervisory manager needs to have a good understanding of and sensitivity towards people, a grasp of the principles of learning and also an interest in what 'makes people tick'. How is this knowledge acquired? It may be that people are chosen to supervise because they already have an intuitive grasp of what is required. However, there is always much to be learned, and this can be done by tapping into learning resources that are readily available in the workplace. Peers, superiors, colleagues and patients are all useful sources of knowledge and understanding about these things. Knowing where to go and who to ask for help in locating knowledge is another useful skill that is required of the supervisory manager.

> Thinking back to Chapters 2 and 3, can you recall instances when you have learned with the purpose of developing skills, understanding, performance and change? Was it easy to locate relevant sources? Who did you go to for help?

Community of practice

In this chapter we have looked at the supervisory manager within a working context peopled by others. At any point in time we are all members of several 'communities', although we may not readily recognise this. For example, at work we may be members of and define ourselves by the multi-disciplinary team that provides a service, or by the professional/vocational group represented by our job title, or by our role as a supervisory manager among the group of supervisory managers. In some communities we will have little or no expertise, and in others we will have a great deal – we may be novices or we may be experts, or somewhere in between. In each community we will have the opportunity to do some learning, and occasionally there will be some conflict of views. The necessity for reconciling varying views of the management role provides an opportunity to learn.

It is rare for anyone to work in complete isolation, but how many people consider the value of using those around them as a source of expertise? The community of managers can provide ideas, challenge, support and novelty to enable further learning – and the whole will undoubtedly be greater than the sum of its parts.

> On being asked how they learned to do their job, people frequently talk about the benefit of asking their colleagues for tips, or watching how other people perform, but would they recognise these as 'sources of expertise'?

Summary

We have moved from a concern with the individual manager and their managing to a picture of the development of skills to manage within the broader context of the workplace community. When we think of the environment within which it is taking place, the complexity of supporting learning in the workplace becomes apparent. Yet in coming to recognise the limits of individual managers and their workplaces as determinants of performance and impact, we have been given an important opportunity to improve our understanding of how managers might support the learning of others.

In the next and subsequent chapters I shall introduce some ideas about the organisational context within which learning is taking place, and consider what helps and what hinders learning. I shall describe a model that can be used as a template to hold up to an organisation (and we shall define this more carefully to suit our purposes) so that we can identify the strong areas and the weak ones where improvement can take place.

Further reading

- Blackler F (1995) Knowledge, knowledge work and organisations: an overview and interpretation. *Organization Stud.* 16: 1021–46.
- Boud D, Keogh R and Walker D (eds) (1985) *Reflection: turning experience into learning.* Kogan Page, London.
- Schein EH (1980) *Organisational Psychology.* Prentice Hall, Englewood Cliffs, NJ.

Chapter 7

Factors that affect workplace learning

Over the last few decades there has been much interest in the way that organisations develop and change, as well as in the significance of the contribution to this, and to the economy generally, made by particular groups. These might include, for example, those working in manufacturing or financial services, or those under the age of 25, or those over the age of 50. Indeed, over the last 20 years, as the UK manufacturing base has shrunk, the following question has been constantly asked, both in the media and elsewhere. Do we need to manufacture goods, or can we buy everything we need from other countries, and can we earn our living by selling our services abroad? And as the age profile of the population has altered, we have seen moves to keep young people in education, and to abolish 'ageism' in the workplace.

Questions such as this are based on an approach that regards people as repositories of 'human capital' – an idea that categorises human input to the economy in a similar way to that of financial capital. This approach rests on the view that the more skills people possess, the greater their productivity will be, and the greater will be their personal reward in the form of money and job satisfaction. Consequently there has also been much interest in the role of motivation in influencing outcomes at work, and in the expectations of workers as learners and their style and level of participation.

Despite the breadth of what has been researched and written, the reality of changing the pattern of working practices is fraught with difficulty, and practical guidance on how this can be achieved is thin on the ground. Among other things, changes are influenced by the environment within which work occurs, including the systems and culture of the workplace. Many writers have contributed to our understanding of these influences. Popular among these have been Peter Senge, who wrote about the 'five disciplines of organisational learning', and Etienne Wenger, who wrote about 'learning communities'. Arguably, however, as understanding is transferred from the university to what goes on in the workplace, something is lost. Translating research into practice is not as straightforward as it might appear.

It is therefore commendable that an organisation of the size and with the profile of the NHS has chosen to attempt what many would see as impossible. Public commitment has been made to the concept of lifelong learning as an aid to workforce flexibility. This approach emphasises the widening of access to learning, and the deepening of roles, as well as creating new opportunities within the existing workforce. Influential policy documents have included the *NHS Plan* (published in 2000) followed by the *NHS Improvement Plan* (published in 2004), as well as the Public Health White Paper *Choosing Health: Making Healthy Choices Easier* (published in December 2004) and, most recently, *Creating a Patient-Led NHS* (published in 2005). Considerable work is in hand to make a reality of the ambitions expressed here. The subtext is that change requires a shift of strategies, skills and structures if the goal of a modern and improved health service is to be achieved.

Lifelong learning (or more accurately *work-long* learning) is a relatively new concept for the NHS, although the phrase was first coined in the 1960s.

According to the Government's Department for Education and Skills:

creating a culture of lifelong learning is crucial to sustaining and maintaining our international competitiveness. Rapid technological and organisational change means that however good initial education and training is, it must be continuously reinforced by further learning throughout working life. This must happen if skills are to remain relevant, individuals as employable and firms able to adapt and compete.

(DfES, 1998: p. 3)

The concept of reflective, experiential learning taking place while working has grown in prominence as it has become acknowledged that we cannot all be constantly absent from work to attend courses. Writers such as Donald Schon, in his seminal text *The Reflective Practitioner*, and Chris Argyris, who wrote about 'single and double loop learning', have had a great deal of influence in promoting and shaping ideas in this field. At the same time we have seen the growth of vocational qualifications, with their emphasis on relevance and ongoing skills development. So the significance of the workplace as a learning environment as well as a working environment has become generally accepted.

The implication of the modernisation agenda

What an organisation becomes emerges from the relationship of its members rather than being determined simply by the global choices of some individuals.

(Stacey, Griffin and Shaw, 2000: p. 52)

Changed ways of doing work in the new economy are the result of influences such as global competition, technological change, changing market regulation and increased consumer sophistication leading to raised expectations. Over the last few decades we have seen many structural changes in organisations, such as the following:

- *outsourcing*, which happened to support services in healthcare during the 1990s and has become established since then
- the *flattening of hierarchies*, led by a number of initiatives, a recent example being the *Agenda for Change*
- *downsizing*, which goes along with outsourcing in an attempt to make efficiency savings
- the *non-standardisation of work*, which tends to occur when teams take collective responsibility for providing a service
- the *breakdown of traditional occupational demarcations* as new roles and responsibilities are created in response to changing circumstances, such as demographic and technological changes.

Modernisation has already resulted in organisations that function with much less bureaucracy than was previously the case. The intention of this has been to allow greater flexibility and shorter response times, and the consequences have been felt in every working environment.

Changes to the way we work are happening constantly, and it often feels as if the pace is increasing. It is unquestionable that *Creating a Patient-Led NHS* (published in 2005), with its emphasis on patient choice and payment by results, will lead to enormous changes in how and where staff work. Employing organisations will also change, and many professionals will find themselves working within different organisational configurations, such as the not-for-profit and private sectors. These changes will have a massive influence on activity. We all – workers and patients alike – have more information at our disposal than ever before, and we are being enabled to use this information to make choices from a broad range of treatments, confident that we are protected by tight regulation to ensure that decisions are optimal. To get from where we are now to where we will be in five years' time will require significant workplace learning.

In order to remain competitive in a globalised world, workers in the UK have to be more knowledgeable, more creative and more innovative than their peers abroad. To the same extent as with other industries, this affects public sector healthcare, where we have seen rising expectations on the part of service users, and drives for efficiency via published targets, all of which require increased knowledge. The majority of jobs in the UK now have a 'skills profile' which lists the competences necessary in order to do the job. Most jobs require qualifications that are current and continuously refreshed because skills have a very short shelf-life. In the NHS, a Knowledge and Skills Framework (KSF) has been developed against which performance is appraised and promotion granted.

Knowledge work and innovation emphasises the practical, and is procedural and interdisciplinary. High-performance working of this kind is very dependent on the context within which it occurs. However, workplaces can be incoherent, and they can lack a structure to support learning, partly because they have outcomes and targets that are wholly specific to the task for which they are created. The question of how we deal with this underpins the approaches described in this part of the book.

Modelling the workplace as a site for learning

I would like to introduce another model. This one is designed to highlight the context within which learning in organisational settings takes place. My reason for looking at the context (or the organisational environment) is to uncover what might help and what might hinder learning – in other words, to uncover the gaps and weaknesses that are revealed by looking closely at what is going on in workplaces. The model is deliberately broad, in that it acknowledges the influence of overarching agendas at play which influence what occurs in workplaces, while at the same time it draws attention to the individual styles, motivations and outcomes of individual learning. However, the focus is mainly on the workplace itself, and the systems, policies and cultures that shape each one as a site for learning.

In presenting this model I want to draw attention to the arrangements in the varying settings within which learning is planned, and the norms and rules that exist there. I am seeking to highlight the intentions and the realities with regard to what *should* happen and what *does* happen. I am also adopting a long-term perspective, to take account of what is happening now, while recognising past and future influences on learning. So my perspective emphasises the cultures and the discourses that take place, that emerge over time and that are ongoing. My focus is on dynamism and evolution rather than on anything that can be considered to be static.

	National	*Organisational*	*Individual*
Investment	Economic	Systems	Processes
Direction	Policy context	Policy intentions	Purpose
Congruence	Socio-political trends	Culture	Disposition

The aim of this model is to focus on the factors that influence work-based learning. I have categorised these factors into three main areas. First, there are the overarching contextual (national) factors that derive from the economic and socio-political situation which can operate in any regime and at any particular time. Different sectors of the economy lay varying emphasis on learning, and this alters over time. Whether public or private, situated in the new or the old economic sector, and dominated by high or low skills, there will be variation in the value that is attached to the importance of learning. There will be differences in the extent to which the population is inclined to view learning as useful and valuable. A decade ago we all assumed that (formal) learning ceased by the time we reached the age of about 22, by which time we had enough knowledge inside us to see us through to retirement. How very different from the 'cradle-to-grave' times in which we now live. For the NHS in the UK these issues are played out in a very public forum, and we have to be mindful of the widespread perceptions of what is appropriate in the circumstances. To a large extent these factors – the economic, the policy environment and the socio-political – are 'given', and although we have to be aware of them, the chances of changing them are very limited, if not impossible.

My second category is somewhat different. Here the concern is with the systems and structures within the specific organisation in which learning is assumed to be taking place. Systems and protocols are generally seen as necessary for the efficient running of any business, and arguably they are also essential for keeping track of learning and development. However, systematisation does not always fulfil the hopes of those who invest time and effort in putting systems in place. Policies that have been made elsewhere have to be implemented within a cultural environment that differs considerably from place to place. Value judgements have to be made about what makes for a positive and 'good' environment for learning, and action must be taken to adjust the parameters that surround everyday activity. So decisions that are made nationally and/or regionally have to be implemented locally, and the result is very variable. However, there is the potential for measurement, evaluation and change within an organisation, allowing the identification of shortfalls or gaps in provision and thus offering the possibility of improvement.

My third category is that which concerns the individual worker/learner. Clearly factors such as preferred processes, purposes and commitment to learning will vary from person to person. However, although awareness of these factors is necessary, it is unlikely that employment itself will be dependent on this, since the priority is unlikely to be recruitment of *good learners* as opposed to *good workers*. Yet this does not mean that these things can be ignored. Attention and creativity can result in improvement and thus lead to a motivated and enthused workforce. Although somewhat secondary, it would be a mistake to regard these factors as entirely 'given'.

My model suggests that in order to understand the circumstances within which workplace learning occurs, we need to look holistically at a number of factors. However, few of us have the power and opportunity to change the economic or political climate that surrounds learning, and we will have only limited opportunity to change our workers/learners, so this leaves us with the workplace itself. If we can identify what it is about workplaces that influences learning, we can make strides in better supporting learning and thus improving healthcare.

Work-related learning is often a 'just-in-time' response to the specific needs of an organisation, but for the individual the purpose of work-related learning may be generalised, longer-term and career driven. Tension between individuals and organisations, with learning caught in the middle, arises when the individual fails to register the significance of the organisational context within which learning is occurring, and the organisation ignores these individual needs. However, I believe that it is useful to consider them together to enable us to examine everyday interaction within organisations and how fertile this might prove to be as a generator of learning.

The organisational context of learning

An organisation becomes what it is because of the systems that its managers design, the actions they take and how they deal with risk – all in a competitive world. What an organisation becomes emerges from the relationship of its members rather than being determined simply by the global choices of some individuals. No two organisational settings are the same, and this must impact on the relationships and the learning of members of those organisations.

Unpacking the organisational factors will allow us to see clearly what does happen and to compare it with what should happen. In the next chapter I shall look at these factors in considerable detail, but for now I shall briefly introduce them. I have categorised them as follows:

- the systems in place
- policy and how it is implemented
- the cultures of the workplace.

Systems

Systems thinking has become the predominant model for reviewing the way in which organisations function. Such an approach draws on the example set by nature, which is recognised as non-random and selective, and which produces optimal results. The systems approach helps to identify connections that have identifiable causes yet are distant in time and location. Knowing what they are can help us to anticipate and illuminate unintended and unexpected consequences, including those connected with human actions. This is clearly a useful way of thinking, and it can be beneficial if we wish to explore the effects of a workplace context on learning.

However, there are significant weaknesses associated with systems thinking that reduce the likely benefits. For example, this approach focuses on *what gets done*, and may therefore miss important features by not paying sufficient attention to *what gets excluded*. In other words, it may overlook (because it doesn't pay attention to) the complexities of organisational life. In reality there is always a gap between what should happen and what in the pressured real world that we inhabit does happen. Managers invariably find that their plans and carefully thought through protocols fall down, and they are left with a situation in which they have to improvise – where they end up 'getting it done anyway', *in spite of* rather than *because of* the systems that are in place – in other words, not the way that they had planned but using some compromise situation. This leaves them feeling inadequate, as if they are in charge but not in control, and this can be detrimental to the work-based learning that is desired and intended. Paying close attention to the rhetoric and the reality of systems and protocols will help us to identify those weak links that hinder learning.

Policy

The direction that learning provision takes is influenced by decisions about policy that are made elsewhere, frequently at national level, and it is well known that priorities are often governed by other imperatives. At the same time, the complex nature of supply and demand within the modern NHS is such that those making decisions about skills needs are often geographically and psychologically distanced from those 'on the ground'. With the growth of commissioning and contracted supply and demand, much policy is now implemented regionally and its effect is felt by large numbers of people. How to reconcile this with the individual employee and his or her personal development needs is a huge challenge.

Theory and observation tell us that learning is a social activity. Ask most people what they do if they have a technical problem and very few will tell you that they first consult the manual. They are much more likely to ask a colleague or to try by trial and error to find a solution. This is sound, pragmatic, non-formal learning, which by definition is lifelong, and which I have described in earlier chapters. It is not based on an agenda decided by others, and it is incidental to doing the job. It can be almost accidental, resulting from activity that wasn't designed or planned specifically to enable learning, but during which recognisable learning has taken place. Conversely, it can be deliberative. Planning to watch and learn how colleagues 'do it' and succeed is a well-known and effective way of learning. However, socially constructed learning of this kind is almost impossible to mandate by policy, although it is unquestionably what is required for improvement of performance and for organisational modernisation and change. How can we reconcile these necessary aspects of workplace learning?

Culture

Professor Chris Argyris wrote powerfully about behavioural systems in organisations, and in particular about the behaviours that result from both formal and informal organisational demands, and the behaviour that results from the individual's attempt to fulfil his or her own needs in the context of those organisational demands. After starting a new job it doesn't take very long to pick up the vibes about such things as dress-code, style of interaction, and which rules can be ignored and which must be followed carefully. And these things can vary a great deal, even within the same company.

Any one organisation can display signs of many different cultures, some of which will be more supportive of learning than others. In all likelihood it is those in which people feel themselves to be part of a supportive community where adaptive learning will be achieved and shared.

The NHS is often seen as bureaucratic and overburdened with rules and regulations. Bureaucracy within any organisation leads to a sense of frustration on the part of many workers, who feel that they have limited influence on the change agenda. In environments where there is also pressure to meet targets, and work is primarily task focused, this can lead to a negative culture that breeds a 'just-in-time' mentality. This is not an environment that is conducive to learning and to sharing learning.

Summary

In this chapter I have shifted the focus to begin to examine healthcare workplaces as environments within which learning can occur. I have suggested that there are 'factors' which can be identified, measured and changed. By improving the environment, we can improve learning and thus we can improve the delivery of healthcare.

In an ideal world an organisation will have a clear understanding of those external and internal national factors – economic and socio-political – which drive it towards change, and which necessitate the development of a vision and the clear articulation of objectives. Systems and protocols that enable sound communication of this to staff will be in place to help each of them to understand their contribution. A supportive organisation can then delegate responsibility to individuals who will, in a co-participatory way and with the self-belief that is born out of the trusting environment within which they work, take up the challenge.

Personally I can't relate this description to any organisation that I have known. This is surprising in view of the enthusiasm and commitment for workplace learning that are expressed by many people. Clearly something is preventing the implementation of intentions about learning. I believe that this 'something' can be found by examining the systems, policy practices and culture in workplaces, and that careful scrutiny of these can uncover problem areas. It is to this subject that we shall turn in the next chapter.

Further reading

- Argyris C (1994) *On Organisational Learning*. Basil Blackwell, Oxford.
- DfES (1998) *The Learning Age: a renaissance for a new Britain*. HMSO, London. www.dfes.gov.uk/publications.
- Schon DA (1983) *The Reflective Practitioner: how professionals think in action*. Basic Books, New York.
- Senge PM (1990) *The Fifth Discipline: the art and practice of the learning organisation*. Doubleday, New York.
- Stacey RD, Griffin D and Shaw P (2000) *Complexity and Management: fad or fact?* Sage Publications, London.
- Wenger E (1998) *Communities of Practice: learning, meaning and identity*. Cambridge University Press, Cambridge.

Chapter 8

The factors explained

Introduction

In Chapter 7 some ideas were introduced about the influences that, over time and from sector to sector, dictate the degree to which learning changes as a priority area for organisations. In thinking about these influences and the way that they impact on work-related learning, I suggested that it is helpful to consider the connections between the investment that is made at national, organisational and individual levels, and the direction that is taken as a result of Government policies. I suggested that within any organisation there are identifiable factors that help or hinder learning; and I also drew attention to factors that influence the extent to which individual employees embrace or reject learning opportunities provided for them. Broadly speaking, this is the framework of my model of 'factors that influence work-related learning'.

In this chapter I want to look more closely at these categories, to prepare for work in Chapters 9 and 10 that will allow us to manipulate and improve the situation in the workplace, and to make our organisation 'ready' for learning. I believe that, although we have to be aware of the national factors and the individual factors, we are not in a position to alter their influence on learning. So although we should be mindful of them, we shall concentrate on the organisational factors, descriptions of which form the basis of this chapter.

The model is designed to help us to make sense of the trends surrounding learning for health improvement. From recent publications I have identified that the main drivers influencing developments around learning for healthcare workers include the following:

- the *quality of the patient experience*
- the *efficiency* with which the service can be provided
- the degree to which *accountability* within roles and responsibilities can be maintained during times of economic, social and technological change
- the *level of job satisfaction* within the changing roles of healthcare workers.

We need to be aware of these drivers as we plan learning, because all of these things will improve the delivery of healthcare. These drivers form the background to all of the recent policy documents that have been published by the Department of Health and other Government departments. In particular, the emphasis on quality of delivery and patient choice has become central to the Government's determination to modernise and improve the delivery of care. With this in mind, what follows is a description of the key factors that influence the effectiveness of work-related formal and non-formal learning in the NHS as these things relate to service improvement.

Organisational factors

Systems and protocols

Factor 1: systematised planning

Planning of future workforce needs has had a chequered history in the UK. The strategy was most actively pursued during the 1970s, developing from the interest engendered by Taylorism and the doctrine of 'scientific management'. This was the era of 'time and motion' and job standardisation – the conviction that every job could be broken down into small routine components which could then be closely managed.

At that time it was believed that skills needs could be predicted with accuracy over a medium- to long-term trajectory, and that young people could be directed towards training to meet future needs with some degree of accuracy. There was also a desire to keep employment levels high by substituting labour for capital investment, and in some industries Government grants were offered to support labour retention at the expense of investment in new machinery. Unfortunately this policy came to grief and led to a period of stagnation because employers followed the rational course of under-investing in infrastructure and over-investing in person power. Over the long term this strategy leads to a slowdown in productivity which will eventually make a company uncompetitive.

Consequently, for many years the idea that skills needs can be predicted with certainty has been unfashionable, but the concept is coming back into favour, with the emphasis now directed more at organisational skills shortages rather than at sectoral-level requirements. However, predictions are only useful if they lead directly to appropriate responses. Large organisations, particularly those that employ a high proportion of human resources such as the NHS, are particularly at risk if workforce planning is done in isolation and without the benefit of accurate information. Healthcare organisations are increasingly investing in learning in parallel with workforce planning. Given the growing scarcity of and increasing competition for workers this makes sense, but there is considerable debate about the effectiveness of this kind of systems thinking at local level.

Government policies to promote skills development have led to the growth of initiatives such as Investors in People, and the output from various management schools has led to the adoption of modern management techniques such as appraisal systems, frequently based on structured competence frameworks. Thus in the NHS we have the Knowledge and Skills Framework, which is used in conjunction with personal development planning to enable organisational future proofing and career pathways for all staff.

However, the success of such approaches relies heavily on those in the front-line who are charged with implementing the systems and protocols that are put in place at senior level. Because managers are only human, there will be variation in the levels of understanding and commitment of those undertaking the tasks implied by the systems approach. Because people and organisations are complex entities, it is almost impossible to consider and plan for every eventuality. And so, despite the great effort invested, systems will never reach perfection or consistency in application.

Factor 1

The organisation, while operating a long-term plan that encompasses all of the workforce, recognises that systematisation has to be approached flexibly.

Factor 2: the way that work is organised

Much learning takes place while people are working, but it does not get recognised as such because it is not given the status of 'codified knowledge' – in other words, it isn't public knowledge and it hasn't been written down somewhere. Yet every time we think about what we are doing and how we might improve next time, some valuable learning occurs. And if we share our experiences with others, this kind of learning becomes doubly useful. The more challenges and variety that we face daily, the greater the number of opportunities there will be for this kind of reflective engagement with work.

However, work is organised in busy healthcare units to maximise efficiency and the execution of tasks. The more experienced the worker, the less deliberation is needed to perform tasks. So the tendency is to encourage specialisation and repetition among workers. Think of the way that we learn to drive a car. At first we are novices and have to think about every stage of switching the engine on, engaging gear, moving off and monitoring other traffic. However, after some practice we get more adept and start to do these things automatically. Eventually we reach expert status when we can drive in every conceivable situation – for example, while having a conversation or planning the weekly shop. Arguably we have learned most and been challenged more in those early stages and, give or take the occasional exceptional circumstance, we will have to diversify (perhaps by driving other vehicles?) in order to continue to learn at the same pace as we did when we were novices. Similarly, in the workplace, if our tasks are routine and repetitive, the opportunities for learning are limited.

But it doesn't have to be that way. Challenges can be planned and organised in order to offer opportunities for learning – to take heed of the needs of each individual as well as those of the organisation. Within the constraints of the need to maintain standards, there are likely to be many opportunities to work alongside a changing number of people from varying professional backgrounds. This can seamlessly lead to learning, especially if people are given time to talk to each other about their experiences. A sympathetic line manager can add value by acting as a sounding-board and giving frequent feedback, but peer-to-peer dialogue is invaluable for promoting learning.

The annual appraisal is the time and place for relevant discussions and exploration of possibilities, but more frequent informal interaction between the individual and his or her line manager can result in ad-hoc and opportunistic learning that is beneficial. However, there is a price to pay for utilising such an approach to learning. In economic circles it is called the 'opportunity cost', and it recognises that if you are doing one thing you have to 'pay' for it by giving up something else. For example, you might want to go to the cinema and also to play tennis, but you can't do both at the same time! Similarly, organising work to accommodate learning will have a 'cost' attached to it, and that cost is measured in hours and minutes.

Factor 2

Work is organised and managed to facilitate non-formal workplace learning.

Factor 3: the role of supervisory managers

No matter what role we fill, we are all supervised in the workplace. In general, the relationship between supervisor and supervised is perceived as unequal and regulatory, but it does not necessarily have to be so. Supervisors can mentor as well as monitor.

It has long been recognised that NHS staff who work in support roles (approximately 40% of the total number of staff) are significantly under-provided with opportunities for education and training. Significant efforts have been made to redress this situation, and good practice in providing learning opportunities is growing in the service, but there are infrastructural issues that prevent expansion, and delivery at scale of a realistic 'skills escalator' for the majority remains a chimera.

However, with the increasing recognition of the value of the workplace as a site for learning, priorities have shifted. Less emphasis is being placed on releasing staff, and more effort is being directed towards developing creative ways of ensuring that staff are encouraged to learn while they are working. Part of this challenge is to ensure that learners are adequately supported, and that appropriate feedback is provided to enable effective and meaningful progression to be made. Although models differ, workplace learning generally requires the learner to take more responsibility for their own advancement. It is often less structured and more ad hoc than learning that takes place in the more conventional setting of a college or training room.

There are a number of advantages to constructing learning close to the everyday experience of working, including greater relevance, consistency and coherence, while moderating the psychological barriers encountered by those who may have had unsuccessful school careers. Collaborative learning through work accentuates the role of peers and line managers in fostering an appropriate learning environment, thereby mitigating some of the negativity of the past.

Supervisory managers have an ongoing responsibility to ensure that those whom they manage are adequately supported, and to ensure that all opportunities to learn are recognised and capitalised upon. In some cases this is part of their formal job description, while in others it is less well recognised. In some professions, such as nursing, there are dedicated posts to support the gaining of practical understanding at work, and those who fill these posts are expected to be qualified facilitators of learning.

Feedback and the sharing of relevant information as a regular component of workplace support have a very positive effect on learning. Collaboration through activity-based teamwork and communities of practice will lead to effective learning as well as efficient practice. This is a time-consuming activity and should therefore be a recognised responsibility within the performance indicators of every supervisory manager. However, the way in which these issues are approached and implemented will vary. Implementation will be influenced by a number of factors, such as organisational context and priorities, the skills of supervisory managers, and the value attached to personal development in organisations.

There is a real need for training and development of middle-management staff to enable them to take on this vital role properly. It is also crucial to make clear the links between learning and the objectives of the organisation – this is as important as providing appropriate resources in the form of time and money.

Factor 3

Supervisory managers play a recognised and significant role in supporting employees for whom they are responsible in order to achieve continual learning.

Policy implementation

Factor 4: varying individual and organisational needs

As the pressure to modernise has gathered pace, the scale and scope of policy making have been dizzying. And the challenge of translating the aims of policy makers into reality has been complicated by continually altering structures within the service. Although everyone involved wants to do their best for patients, it is very difficult to keep abreast of new developments. This is true for all aspects of healthcare delivery, including the learning element that is concomitant with improvement.

The direction that learning provision 'on the ground' takes is influenced by decisions about policy that are made elsewhere, generally at national level, and it is acknowledged that priorities are frequently governed by imperatives other than those felt at local level. The complex nature of supply and demand within the modern NHS is such that those who make decisions about skills needs are often geographically and psychologically distanced from those in the front-line. With the growth of strategic health authorities, workforce development directorates and contracted supply and demand, much policy is implemented regionally, and its effect is felt by large numbers of people. How can this be reconciled with the individual trust or primary care trust employee and his or her personal development needs?

Within the organisation, the bridge between these two groups is the training and development capacity within the HR directorate and the supervisory manager. Here attempts are made to recognise and reconcile varying needs, but arguably organisational requirements are short-term and skills focused, whereas individual needs are likely to be more long-term, broader and career (rather than skills) oriented. HR policy at organisational level seeks to accommodate these sometimes conflicting requirements. Creative thinking should make it possible for local policy to build in opportunities for individual career development while at the same time ensuring that the needs of the employing organisation are met.

This is the national ambition, but is it the local goal?

Factor 4

Policy about future workforce planning takes both individual and organisational learning needs into account.

Factor 5: policy concerning formal and non-formal learning

Both theory and observation tell us that learning is a social activity. As was mentioned earlier, if you ask most people what they do if they have a technical problem, very few will tell you that they go first to the manual.

They are more likely to ask a colleague or to try to find a solution by trial and error. Ask most people how they learned to do the job and you will rarely hear anyone say 'I learned it on a course and here's my certificate to prove it'. They are more likely to say 'by being thrown in at the deep end' or 'by watching colleagues do it'.

These are perfectly valid forms of learning. Ideally, though, to gain the maximum benefit from this kind of shared learning, the environment of the workplace should provide opportunities and support. The context within which learning takes place is crucially either a help or a hindrance.

When planning staffing levels and skills mix it must be recognised that learning has resource implications. This primarily means time to challenge, to reflect, to make and rectify mistakes, to learn and to share experiences. Staff and common rooms, and an informal culture based on 'corridor conversations', are great sites for learning.

We are talking here about non-formal learning, which by definition is lifelong, is not based on an agenda decided by others, and is incidental to doing the job. It can be serendipitous or deliberative – coincidental or planned. Building on both personal experience and that of others means that the level of understanding reached is greater than that of each individual learner.

Team structures are important in healthcare working environments, but the fact that teams learn together and from each other while working together is often overlooked. Variations in team relationships, functions and responsibilities offer a range of learning possibilities, and this should be capitalised on wherever possible.

It is generally recognised that such approaches are beneficial, but the reality is that policy to support non-formal as well as formal learning is very difficult to implement, given the plethora of pressures faced in modern workplaces.

Factor 5

Policy takes into account the creation of non-formal as well as formal learning opportunities in a social setting to enable sharing of experience.

Factor 6: the variety of support mechanisms

How often financial solutions seem to provide a 'quick fix' for problems with staff – a training course can appear to be the most effective response to intractable skills problems. And of course there are situations where a course can offer an appropriate means of plugging skills gaps – but it shouldn't stop there.

Policy that encourages psychological support is part of the equation, too. This is about reinforcement, about sending signals that learning is an approved activity and offering support from various quarters – from director level, from local line manager level and from peer group level. Custom and practice have to reflect this, and intentions have to be talked about and followed through so far as learning is concerned. And it is about celebrating success.

An appropriate location for learning takes the workplace into account, but should be backed by a generously equipped resource centre. How many training departments are housed in basements and Portakabins? And what does that convey about the value which is placed on learning? Materials frequently vary from the adequate, up to date and cared for to the dog-eared and ancient.

Technology-supported learning is becoming commonplace – less so the level of support offered. Are computers readily available or locked away? Is 'technology' confined to the occasional CD-ROM or does it mean multiple approaches, some of which might be experimental and therefore risky? Do people have access outside working hours? Do they have protected learning time?

National policy is designed to include provision for adequate support for all learners, but making a reality of this ambition is tough, especially when it is recognised that support takes varying forms, ranging from financial to psychological, infrastructural and technological. Significantly, it has to be recognised that learning is a time-consuming process, and that it involves the making of mistakes that provide opportunities for further learning. It is especially beneficial if mistakes can be articulated and shared in a non-confrontational way, so that the learning possibilities are increased across the organisation.

Policy infers that support should be offered, but the reality is that support is patchy in most organisations, primarily because of the costs and the wide range of needs encountered at ground level.

Factor 6

Policy includes support in financial, psychological, infrastructural and technological forms to ensure that learning opportunities are maximised.

Culture

Factor 7: rigid rules and bendable rules

Organisational culture is generally difficult to pin down when you are there in the midst of it, but is clearly apparent from the outside. Culture is about the expectations that people bring to work, how they behave and interact with each other, the spoken and unspoken rules that exist, and knowing which of these have to be obeyed to the letter and which are adaptable. We know about dress code and who speaks to whom – what can be said and what is best left unsaid. Culture is also about whether we can admit to mistakes – and who we can admit them to – or whether we endeavour to pass the buck at the first opportunity. How do we know these things? They are not usually part of the induction programme! In fact they are rarely spoken about, but after joining an organisation it doesn't take very long before one begins to understand what is tolerated and what isn't.

As early as 1960 Professor Chris Argyris was writing about behavioural systems in organisations. He talked about the behaviours that result from both formal and informal organisational demands, and the behaviour that results from the individual's attempts to fulfil his or her own needs in the context of those organisational demands.

The NHS is often portrayed as bureaucratic, overburdened with rules and regulations. Bureaucracy within any organisation leads to a sense of frustration on the part of many workers, who feel that they have a limited influence on the change agenda. In environments where there is also pressure to meet targets, and work is primarily task focused, this can lead to a negative culture that breeds a 'just-in-time' mentality.

Is it possible to make a realistic assessment of an organisation's culture? Can weaknesses and limitations be confronted, to be used as a platform for further learning? Can rhetoric and spin be avoided, and efforts continually made to ensure that the culture is one of openness and sharing, with attention paid to individual experiences that impact on working life? It would be good to think so – that modernisation involves a true confrontation of necessary change, and a willingness to get involved in positive cultural engagement.

What is held up as appropriate in terms of relationships and working practice should correlate closely with what happens in practice. Rules and regulations should be kept to a minimum and unnecessary strictures avoided. This is the intention behind current changes that stress the need for collaboration, efficiency and putting the patient first. The overall culture should ideally strive for the creation of a community rather than focus on bureaucratic procedures, but how close are most organisations to this ideal?

Factor 7

Organisational culture fosters openness and sharing rather than hierarchy and bureaucracy.

Factor 8: the power of communication

In some countries, if people at work are engrossed in conversation it is assumed that they are discussing a work-related issue. In the UK there is a tendency to assume that they are discussing last night's episode of *Big Brother*. In many NHS organisations there are established patterns based on custom and practice of who can talk to whom, and about what. Hierarchical imperatives require that junior staff generally do not speak to senior staff about anything other than the most formal work-related issues, or that communication across professional boundaries is non-existent. This leads to particular patterns of understanding about how the organisation functions, and a level of shared understanding that is very limited.

The *NHS Plan* (published in 2000) stated that:

> *old-fashioned demarcations between staff mean some patients see a procession of health professionals – often recounting the same details to the GP, practice nurse, hospital booking clerk, hospital nurse, care assistant, therapist, junior doctor, and consultant. Information is not shared and investigations are often repeated.*

Despite all the effort, has the situation changed much since then? Equally:

> *unnecessary boundaries exist between the professions which hold back staff from fulfilling their true potential. Three-quarters of house officers do two or more basic tasks not specifically requiring medical training. Up to 40% of patients seeing an orthopaedic consultant in outpatients would be better off being treated by a trained physiotherapist in the first instance. These practices frustrate staff and cause long waits for patients.*

It would be so much more satisfactory if communication patterns were inclusive, supporting a culture of openness rather than obstructing it. Power structures, restrictive practices and knowledge hoarding shouldn't be tolerated in everyday relationships in this present age of informality and knowledge management. The trouble is, most people would agree with this, but still we see no change in the way that professionals behave.

Very few people outside of work would subscribe to a situation where communication is limited to those of equal rank and status, so why does it continue to occur in the workplace? Co-operation and collaborative working practices, coupled with flexibility and creativity in defining and performing job roles, could result in an atmosphere of shared endeavour. Time could then be set aside for useful communication to occur, and infrastructure could be put in place to support this. Efforts could then be made on a continual basis to ensure that improvements continue and are built in, to the benefit of all stakeholders in the healthcare environment.

> **Factor 8**
>
> Communication is recognised as a necessary part of working and learning, and ongoing efforts to encourage this are considered important.

Factor 9: the importance of shared values

In his book entitled *Understanding Organisational Behaviour*, Chris Argyris drew attention to the fact that there are differing outcomes when there is a gap between 'espoused theory' (what we say we do) and 'theory in use' (what we actually do). We are all guilty of some self-deception – convincing others of our concern for the environment while climbing into the 4 × 4 for a trip to the shops. Organisations are no less guilty in this respect. It would be harsh to say that this is always calculated – in fact there is often a lack of awareness of the gap between intentions and actions.

The NHS was set up within the context of a strong set of values regarding what was appropriate activity for the State, and where welfare might contribute to economic performance and the creation of a better life for all members of society. These values are still cited to justify the model of funding and provision of healthcare in the UK. However, with the introduction of increasing private-sector involvement and competition within the service, it is becoming doubtful whether the espoused theory of politicians correlates with their theory in use. What does it look like at the front-line? And how much of this value system is complemented by appropriate education and training provision?

Values are difficult to see and to pin down. And rarely do we articulate our value system to others. More often we assume that everyone is thinking alike about the big issues. Therefore the extent to which we have agreement and harmony about what might be required for good healthcare provision becomes assumed rather than stated.

The way that the NHS sees itself as an organisation and how this is communicated to staff has a significant impact on learning. Metaphors can be a useful means of conveying ideas that are difficult to articulate in other ways, but in order to have meaning they need to be realistic and appropriate. The workplace as a machine with inputs and outputs, with targets and rating scales, and with a constant need to defend its performance against hostile outside forces is unlikely to provide a supportive environment for learning. However, the workplace as a community, with support and guidance freely offered and taken, is more likely to result in employees who feel positively inclined to learn.

> **Factor 9**
>
> The organisation adheres to espoused values that are designed to promote learning.

Summary

In this chapter I have looked very closely at certain aspects of organisations in terms of their environment for learning. In doing so I have tried to draw attention to the potential shortfalls and weaknesses embedded in each factor that might be influential when it comes to learning. In the following chapters I am going to invite you to look closely at your own organisation in order to discover its strengths and weaknesses. Only by doing this can we hope to improve healthcare delivery.

To conclude, I believe that the factors which influence workplace learning can be summarised as follows.

- **Factor 1:** The organisation, while operating a long-term plan that encompasses all of the workforce, recognises that systematisation has to be approached flexibly.
- **Factor 2:** Work is organised and managed to facilitate non-formal workplace learning.
- **Factor 3:** Supervisory managers play a recognised and significant role in supporting employees for whom they are responsible in order to achieve continual learning.
- **Factor 4:** Policy about future workforce planning takes both individual and organisational learning needs into account.
- **Factor 5:** Policy takes into account the creation of non-formal as well as formal learning opportunities in a social setting to enable sharing of experience.
- **Factor 6:** Policy includes support in financial, psychological, infrastructural and technological forms to ensure that learning opportunities are maximised.
- **Factor 7:** Organisational culture fosters openness and sharing rather than hierarchy and bureaucracy.
- **Factor 8:** Communication is recognised as a necessary part of working and learning, and ongoing efforts to encourage this are considered important.
- **Factor 9:** The organisation adheres to espoused values that are designed to promote learning.

Further reading

- Argyris C and Schon DA (1974) *Theory in Practice: increasing professional effectiveness*. Jossey Bass, San Francisco, CA.
- Argyris C and Schon DA (1978) *Organisational Learning: a theory of action perspective*. Addison-Wesley, Reading, MA.
- Department of Health (2000) *The NHS Plan: a plan for investment, a plan for reform*. The Stationery Office, London. www.dh.gov.uk/publications.

Chapter 9

Putting the factors to work

In the last chapter I introduced nine factors that I believe are influential in promoting workplace learning for health improvement. However, awareness of the factors is not enough. In this chapter and the next I would like to help you to put them to work, to examine the extent to which your workplace is supportive of learning. I have devised an approach in a series of steps that will lead to a judgement of effectiveness, and then a plan for improvement. To make the process more transparent I will also provide a worked example, which will take you through the experience of one supervisory manager – Chris Brown – as s(he) identifies and then plans for change in the organisation for which s(he) is responsible.

Using the Learning Web

There are five stages in this section, which take you through all the procedures necessary to learn the effective use of this tool, which is designed to highlight the learning context of an organisation. Each stage contains the following:

- a set of instructions
- a set of explanatory notes
- the forms and diagrams you require
- an example of how to use the procedure.

The instructions are very brief and offer a quick reference to enable you to become familiar with the process. The explanatory notes give further help and offer some background information on the procedures. If you find any of the instructions difficult to follow, carefully read through the example first, which is designed to give a simple illustration of how to use the technique in practice.

Stages 1 and 2: a reality check

Instructions

- Define precisely what you mean by the term 'organisation'.
- Consider the way in which systems, policy and culture are arrived at in this organisation.
- Review the factors with their accompanying indicators.

Explanatory notes

The first part of our process is designed to establish the credibility of the factors. Below you will find the first two steps in the five-stage process that will enable you to assess the effectiveness of your organisational workplace. You will be invited to review the factors that my research has shown are significant, and you will be able to rate your organisation as an environment that promotes work-related learning. This exercise can be usefully done with colleagues, as discovering differences in points of view is a great start to learning!

Listed are the key factors that influence workplace learning, followed by a set of measurable indicators that illustrate each factor. The way in which they are presented will enable you to rate your own organisation, but before doing so you should ask yourself what you mean by 'organisation'. Do you want to examine the NHS in total? In principle this could be done, but for the purposes of this exercise it is probably most useful to think in terms of an independent decision-making entity. This could be a trust or a primary care trust, or it could be a department, ward or GP practice. Size is less relevant than capacity to make decisions about learning and carry them out. Your definition of 'organisation' may be shaped by the breadth of the colleagues or partners whom you include in the discussion.

When you have made your decision, record it here and explain why you chose this particular definition of the term 'organisation'.

Definition of 'organisation':

Reviewing the factors

Now that you have decided what most appropriately represents the concept of 'organisation' for you, you need to consider how to rate your organisation in terms of the following factors, guided by the indicators that accompany them.

Definition of rating classifications:

1 Not applicable
2 Barely applicable
3 Broadly applicable
4 Applicable
5 100% applicable

Factor 1

The organisation, while operating a long-term plan that encompasses all of the workforce, recognises that systematisation has to be approached flexibly.

Indicators

- The organisation has published a strategy for education and skills development and made provision for monitoring of progress.
- There is a clear linkage between this strategy and individual development plans.
- Education and training strategy action plans, once published, are implemented creatively.
- The learning strategy is linked to the organisation's business plan and meets national targets.
- Job descriptions for all staff identify learning responsibilities and accountabilities.
- Everyone in the organisation has equal resource access.
- There are effective mentoring systems in place and in use.
- Audit of personal development plans/appraisals is conducted on an annual basis, and reports are made available to staff.

1 ☐   2 ☐   3 ☐   4 ☐   5 ☐

Please tick the box which most closely describes the current situation in your chosen organisation.

Factor 2

Work is organised and managed to facilitate non-formal workplace learning.

Indicators

- An implementation plan is published identifying a diverse range of learning opportunities (e.g. mentorship, clinical supervision, critical incident review).
- Procedures for facilitating shared learning are established and implemented.
- Supervision is provided for individuals and groups to improve awareness of learning opportunities.
- Protected time is allocated to team and individual learning sessions.
- Formal and informal appraisals are carried out routinely.
- Skills-based training is supported by supervision and assessment of performance in the workplace.

1 ☐   2 ☐   3 ☐   4 ☐   5 ☐

Please tick the box which most closely describes the current situation in your chosen organisation.

Factor 3

Supervisory managers play a recognised and significant role in supporting employees for whom they are responsible in order to achieve continual learning.

Indicators

- Appraisal focuses on learning needs and links this with performance management.
- Responsibility for the learning of others is a component of management development programmes.
- Support is provided for managers to develop their skills and knowledge to support staff learning.
- Support mechanisms exist for managers (e.g. via learning sets and collaborative strategies).
- Formal mechanisms exist for managers/supervisors to meet staff before and after learning events.
- A framework for recording supervision is available and used.

1 ☐   2 ☐   3 ☐   4 ☐   5 ☐

Please tick the box which most closely describes the current situation in your chosen organisation.

Factor 4

Policy about future workforce planning takes both individual and organisational learning needs into account.

Indicators

- Service delivery strategies are linked to patient needs.
- Organisational development needs are linked to patient-focused delivery strategies through service delivery plans.
- Individual learning needs are analysed and aggregated at team/organisation levels.
- Workforce plans are linked to epidemiological evidence.
- All of the above are integrated.
- Clear career pathways are published and there is evidence of successful progress by individuals.
- Education, learning and training frameworks reflect a 'skills escalator' approach and provide accredited programmes for all staff.

1 ☐   2 ☐   3 ☐   4 ☐   5 ☐

Please tick the box which most closely describes the current situation in your chosen organisation.

Factor 5

Policy takes into account the creation of non-formal as well as formal learning opportunities in a social setting to enable sharing of experience.

Indicators

- Policy gives equal time to non-formal and formal learning.
- Induction programmes ensure that staff are informed of the benefits/expectations with regard to learning and sharing.
- Job descriptions include responsibility for sharing learning.
- Resources and facilities for non-formal learning are provided (e.g. learning logs, meeting space, mentorship, etc.).
- Protected learning time is embedded in staff establishments and rotas.
- Regular 'away-days'/residentials to facilitate non-formal learning are provided for all staff.

1 ☐   2 ☐   3 ☐   4 ☐   5 ☐

Please tick the box which most closely describes the current situation in your chosen organisation.

Factor 6

Policy includes support in financial, psychological, infrastructural and technological forms to ensure that learning opportunities are maximised.

Indicators

- All staff have equal access to IT.
- All staff have equal access to library and information services.
- All staff have equal access to learning mentors.
- All staff have equal access to learning spaces.
- All staff have individual email addresses and Internet access.
- Policy on equal access to learning opportunities and evidence of monitoring is available for scrutiny and monitoring.
- There are designated (and ring-fenced) training budgets.
- PCs are available and used in accessible places (e.g. the canteen).
- Training in the use of health/social care databases (integral with induction) is available.

1 ☐   2 ☐   3 ☐   4 ☐   5 ☐

Please tick the box which most closely describes the current situation in your chosen organisation.

Factor 7

Organisational culture fosters openness and sharing rather than hierarchy and bureaucracy.

Indicators

- There is a range of opportunities available for dialogue (e.g. team briefing, open forums, graffiti walls, staff council).
- Dialogue is two-way, honest and taken seriously.
- There are open lines of communication to senior management which are sanctioned and confidential.
- The organisational culture seeks to develop managers to fulfil roles in transformational rather than transactional ways.
- Sharing information and listening to others is promoted by the example of senior managers.
- Questioning and critique of conventions is encouraged.
- Promotion of customer care is one of the cultural expectations that are placed on staff.
- Formal 'learning-from-mistakes' procedures are in place and are evaluated regularly.

1 ☐   2 ☐   3 ☐   4 ☐   5 ☐

Please tick the box which most closely describes the current situation in your chosen organisation.

Factor 8

Communication is recognised as a necessary part of working and learning, and ongoing efforts to encourage this are considered important.

Indicators

- An 'open-door' policy is operated across the organisation.
- The results of surveys are made available to staff.
- Survey results form the basis of local policy changes, which are then evaluated.
- Audit and evaluation outcomes are published.
- Training to enable managers to understand their impact on others is scheduled and obligatory.
- Patient-centred rather than system-centred communication is the norm.
- There are opportunities to share and debrief following learning opportunities.
- The organisation creates a culture in which individuals can communicate the needs of the patient to colleagues openly.

1 ☐   2 ☐   3 ☐   4 ☐   5 ☐

Please tick the box which most closely describes the current situation in your chosen organisation.

Factor 9

The organisation adheres to clearly and publicly stated values that are designed to promote learning.

Indicators

- The organisational mission statement and individual learning portfolios are recognisably co-terminous.
- Appraisal interviews include assessment against the values of both individuals and the organisation.
- Branding of the NHS as a learning and development culture is aggressively pursued.

1 ☐   2 ☐   3 ☐   4 ☐   5 ☐

Please tick the box which most closely describes the current situation in your chosen organisation.

Stages 1 and 2: worked examples

To aid our understanding of the process we are employing here, I now provide a worked example.

The organisation

Chris Brown has been employed for six months as a training manager at Northsouth Primary Care Trust. The demographic spread of the PCT is varied, taking in large rural expanses with problems of accessibility, but also including some significant areas of urban social deprivation. Resources are tight and budgets are subject to fluctuation in line with the requirement to meet a number of urgent financial priorities.

The PCT was part of the second wave to be established, and was made up from a number of practices that had not worked together before. Over the last few years more and more financial and operational responsibilities have fallen to the PCT, and delivery targets are tight. The PCT's management is keen to develop staff as fully as possible, and recognises the need to keep them thoroughly up to date with all new clinical, technical and socio-political changes. However, like most PCTs it also needs to make the most of limited budgets for training and development.

Northsouth PCT wants to be innovative and responsive to new ideas in line with what is happening across the wider NHS agenda. It recognises that this means developing foresight and sensitivity to the needs of staff in order to attract and retain the best available in the region.

The job

Chris's job essentially consists of acting as a consultant in learning, understanding what training needs exist or might exist in the near future, and finding the most appropriate way of meeting those needs. This may include developing training programmes on behalf of different groups of staff, and it occasionally involves delivering short courses in core skills (e.g. assertiveness, time management).

Chris is part of a team consisting of two managers and an administrator, all of whom report through an Executive Director to the PCT Board. Because Chris operates across a range of teams, s(he) needs to be aware of how they fit together, where there might be common needs and where there might be internal expertise that can be exploited.

As Chris travels from team to team, s(he) has become increasingly aware that there is some variation in the way that training is taken up and transferred back to the working environment.

- Some managers seem to encourage staff to learn, while others don't.
- Some workplaces seem to be alive with enthusiastic staff sharing new ideas that have been gained on courses, while others seem to be impervious to change.

- Some workplaces seem to be eager to try out different ways of operating, while others seem to be reluctant to do this.

Of course it's always been the case that workplaces differ, but Chris has started to wonder whether the learning opportunities offered to staff can influence the situation, by encouraging better staff relationships and a more motivated and committed workforce in the less successful units.

Definition of 'organisation':

West Central GP Practice – a small practice with two partners housed in an adapted Victorian terraced house in an outer suburb of a market town.

Staff – a practice manager and one practice nurse, part-time health visitors and district nurses, two receptionists and two full-time GPs.

Busy practice in an area of considerable social deprivation.

Very cramped accommodation – part-timers do not meet unless by arrangement.

Reviewing the factors

Chris has considered the factors and has arrived at the following rating.

Factor 1

The organisation, while operating a long-term plan that encompasses all of the workforce, recognises that systematisation has to be approached flexibly.

1 ☑ 2 ☐ 3 ☐ 4 ☐ 5 ☐

Factor 2

Work is organised and managed to facilitate non-formal workplace learning.

1 ☐   2 ☑   3 ☐   4 ☐   5 ☐

Factor 3

Supervisory managers play a recognised and significant role in supporting employees for whom they are responsible in order to achieve continual learning.

1 ☐   2 ☑   3 ☐   4 ☐   5 ☐

Factor 4

Policy about future workforce planning takes both individual and organisational learning needs into account.

1 ☑   2 ☐   3 ☐   4 ☐   5 ☐

Factor 5

Policy takes into account the creation of non-formal as well as formal learning opportunities in a social setting to enable sharing of experience.

1 ☐   2 ☐   3 ☑   4 ☐   5 ☐

Factor 6

Policy includes support in financial, psychological, infrastructural and technological forms to ensure that learning opportunities are maximised.

1 ☐   2 ☐   3 ☑   4 ☐   5 ☐

Factor 7

Organisational culture fosters openness and sharing rather than hierarchy and bureaucracy.

1 ☐   2 ☑   3 ☐   4 ☐   5 ☐

Factor 8

Communication is recognised as a necessary part of working and learning, and ongoing efforts to encourage this are considered important.

1 ☑   2 ☐   3 ☐   4 ☐   5 ☐

Factor 9

The organisation adheres to espoused values that are designed to promote learning.

1 ☐   2 ☐   3 ☐   4 ☑   5 ☐

Summary

In this chapter we have started the process of audit of the environment for learning that was introduced in Chapter 8. The success of this exercise depends to a great extent on your choice of 'organisation' for scrutiny. Note that, in our worked example, Chris chose to look at a small unit – just one GP practice chosen from the number that made up the PCT. Chris accepted that if changes could be made in one practice, they would provide evidence that s(he) could demonstrate to others. An incremental approach such as this one has more likelihood of success than trying to change everything rapidly.

So far, then, we have chosen the workplace to be audited and we have rated it in terms of the factors that will influence learning. It can be very revealing to do this exercise with colleagues, because it is unlikely that agreement will be reached in the first attempt at rating. However, such differences of opinion can provide a healthy environment for discussion, uncovering assumptions that may never have been tested.

This process can be used in a number of ways. It can be used to compare and contrast two parts of the same organisation (e.g. two wards or two departments), to compare the situation over time (e.g. to find out how things may have changed over a year or so), or to examine the ideal situation compared with the reality of day-to-day goings-on in the organisation.

Now that we have rated our organisation, we need to move on to look at where its strengths and weaknesses lie. This is the focus of the next chapter.

Chapter 10

Planning for change

If you have followed the process described in the previous chapter, you will have undertaken the first two stages of the five-stage process that I introduced in Chapter 9. You should have done the following:

- stage 1 – defined what you mean by 'organisation' for the purposes of audit
- stage 2 – rated your organisation as an environment for workplace learning.

This is a useful exercise in itself, as it will have encouraged you to reflect on how your organisation works and to think more widely about the factors that influence learning in that organisation. You may have done the rating individually or you may have completed it in collaboration with colleagues (the latter approach generally serves as a valuable stimulus for discussion). Now I want to help you to convert this assessment into a form that can be used for further analysis and the drawing up of an action or development plan for your organisation. We shall cover the final three stages of the process, which can be summarised as follows:

- stage 3 – mapping your organisation
- stage 4 – defining a critical factor for improvement
- stage 5 – drawing up a development plan to improve the critical factor.

Stage 3: mapping your organisation

Instructions

- For each factor on the Web diagram plot your rating.
- Join up the rating points to show your diagnosis of the unit as a site for learning.

Explanatory notes

The Organisational Web is a visual tool that I have developed for use in analysis and discussion of learning or personal skills factors. It has three additional benefits to the written ratings scale you have just completed:

1 It provides a single, easy-to-understand visual summary of your assessment.

2 It provides a picture of your organisation's 'profile' in terms of the key factors, which can be compared with the profiles created by other people, or for other organisations.
3 It can be used as a form of 'gap' analysis, to compare current perform-ance with desired target performance.

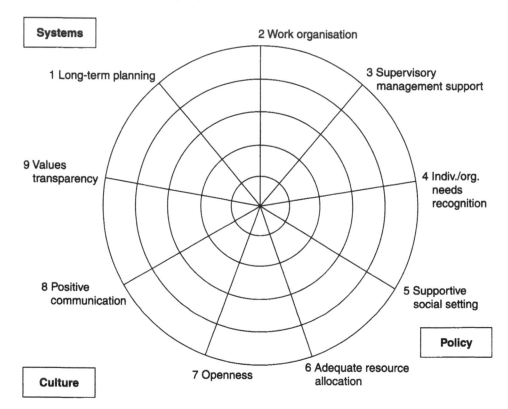

Figure 10.1 The Organisational Web.

Each 'spoke' on the Web represents one of the nine key factors, and each 'circle' represents a rating level, ranging from 1 (the smallest, inner circle) to 5 (the largest, outer circle). Creating your first Web diagram is simply a matter of transferring the scores from your ratings scales on to the appropriate points on the Web. When you have done this, a simple visual 'profile' can be created by joining the points together.

The Web profile can then be used as suggested above. For example, you may wish to ask other colleagues in your organisation to produce individual versions of the Web. These can then be compared as a stimulus for discussion of relative perceptions of performance, or perhaps to help highlight particularly good or bad areas of performance. Similarly, you may want to work with colleagues from another organisation – or from a significantly different part of your own organisation – in order to compare good or bad practice in different environments. In a larger group, a simple way of doing this is by creating Web diagrams on overhead transparencies, which can then be physically overlaid to highlight differences in assessment. A particularly revealing way of using the Web is to draw one that represents the situation before and after (perhaps two years ago compared with now, or now compared with where you want to be in two years' time).

Stage 3: worked example

This is what Chris made of the factors when applied to the Web format (*see* Figure 10.2).

Systems factors

If the unit is to achieve its potential as a site for learning, it needs sound systems and protocols in place to support the activity. Some of these are devolved from the PCT and/or the Department of Health via the NHS, and match quite closely the systems in place at other units. However, on reflection Chris realises that it's not so much the formal acquisition of systems that is important as the way in which they are implemented. Here lies the difference between a workplace that has a positive support role for learning, and one that does not.

Policy factors

Again, most policy initiatives come from external sources and apply to all units in the PCT. However, awareness of what is current, and the extent to which opportunities offered by policy changes are exploited, differ from unit to unit. So Chris is able to form a judgement about this particular unit and to rate it in terms of the factors.

Culture factors

There is wide variation in culture across the various units that make up the PCT. As Chris travels around s(he) can easily see where people form a close-knit community that provides mutual assistance and where they don't. In the case of the unit under consideration, the fact that part-time staff do not meet on an informal basis clearly influences the manner in which they communicate and learn from each other.

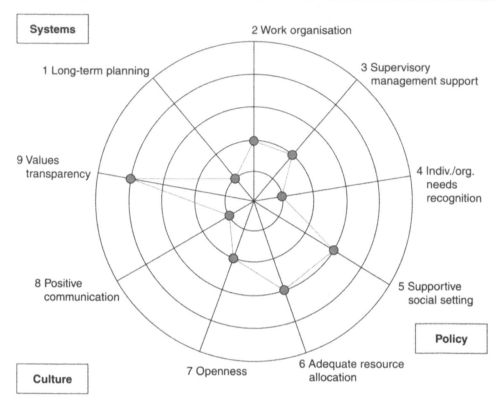

Figure 10.2 The Organisational Web: worked example.

Stage 4: defining a critical factor for improvement

Having a visual representation such as that described above is useful, but there are further steps to be taken.

Instructions

- For each factor on your Web, decide what would be the optimal point.
- Shade the area between 'current' and 'optimal' to give a clearer picture of where the greatest gap lies.
- Think about your priorities for development.

Explanatory notes

The outcome of analysis and discussion using the Web should be a better appreciation of which key factors may offer positive examples of good practice and which may need improvement. In addressing the latter, you may wish to start by deciding what your targets will be. This can be done by returning to the factors and completing the rating scales in terms of desired performance rather than actual perceived performance. Of course it may be tempting to say 'We ought to be "5" on everything', but it is much more helpful to take a realistic view of what is *necessary and achievable*, rather than what is ideal. You may decide, for example, that on factor 8 ('Communication is recognised as a necessary part of working and learning, and ongoing efforts to encourage this are considered important') the physical or time constraints in your part of the NHS mean that communication will always be a problem, and that therefore your realistic target would be an improvement from 2 to 3, or from 3 to 4.

Creating a Web for your target performance permits a simple visual comparison with your assessment of actual performance, as the 'gaps' between actual and target performance can be immediately identified, displayed and compared. Again the process works well as the focus for a group discussion, and may form the starting point for identifying one or more factors for improvement and a strategy for achieving that improvement.

Stage 4: worked example

Figure 10.3 shows that Chris's estimation of the gap between current and optimal performance is close for some factors, but there are obvious priority areas that might be addressed. The following areas stand out as requiring development:

- factor 1 – long-term planning
- factor 4 – taking individual and organisational needs into account
- factor 8 – positive communication.

Chris decides that long-term planning needs to be given priority, since lack of support in this area seems to be causing particular problems at the moment and, due to ever tighter training budgets, it is essential that this situation is improved to enable the unit to work better.

Stage 5: drawing up a development plan to improve the critical factor

Instructions

- Decide on the most appropriate development route.
- Set targets and timescales for yourself, and decide what evidence of improvement you will seek.

Explanatory notes

The final step in the process is to produce a plan of action in order to address the 'gaps' between actual and target performance. Like other organisational goals it is best to make any objectives you set **SMART** (i.e. Specific, Measurable, Achievable, Realistic and Time-bound). A development plan should therefore focus on a relatively small number of factors

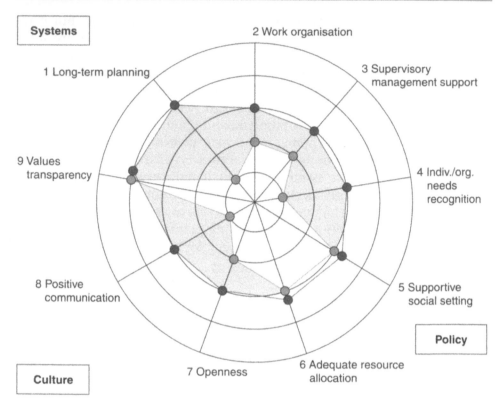

Figure 10.3 The Organisational Web: worked example.

and, within each factor, a realistic number of indicators. As suggested above, levels of improvement should be achievable rather than ideal. There should be clear indications of the actions to be taken, who is responsible for those actions, and the time-frame within which the objectives should be achieved.

Stage 5: worked example

Having decided that an improvement in factor 1 is both a priority and an achievable aspiration, Chris draws up a development plan for achieving goals in relation to this factor. The first step is to return to the full explanation of the factor and the list of measurable indicators. Chris reviews these again in the light of his/her organisation and selects three of the indicators for attention. The achievement of these indicators will be the route to bringing about the desired improvement in work-related learning. Each indicator needs to be measurable, so that if each of these targets is achieved then it would be reasonable to say that the performance rating on this factor has improved from 1 to 4.

Having chosen specific, measurable and achievable targets, the next step is to set a time-frame. Chris decides that two of the three indicators would be achieved within three months, but that realistically it would take six months to achieve the third indicator. S(he) draws up a simple development plan, specifying the main factor, listing the three indicators and putting a target date against each. Chris will also want to include evidence that the targets have been achieved to ensure that they are really measurable.

Finally, Chris needs to consider who else in the organisation will need to be involved in the plan if the targets are to be achieved. Some of these people may be directly involved in its implementation, some may be key stakeholders whose approval will be needed, and some may simply need to be informed of the actions that are being taken. Chris adds these names to the development plan to produce a basic guide for the learning improvement project.

Development plan

Issue to be addressed:

Factor 1
The organisation, while operating a long-term plan that encompasses all of the workforce, recognises that systematisation has to be approached flexibly.

Indicators

- There is a clear linkage between the organisation's strategy and its training and development plans.
- Job descriptions for all staff identify learning responsibilities and accountabilities.
- Audit of personal development plans/appraisals is conducted on an annual basis and reports are made available to staff.

Route

- Consultation with the stakeholders at the practice.
- Agreement with the PCT Board.
- Trial planning document to be drawn up and agreed (to include plan for annual evaluation of progress).

Target

Long-term plan to be agreed, implemented, evaluated, revised, routinely implemented and reviewed.

Time-frame

- Consultation with stakeholders – 3 months.
- Agree document – 6 months.
- Implementation – 6 to 9 months.
- Evaluation and revision – 12 months.

Stakeholders

- All team members of GP practice.
- Executive Director and Board of PCT.
- Strategic Health Authority.

Evidence

- Documentation creating a clear audit trail.
- Systems and protocols in place.
- Evidence of implementation, including personal development plans for all staff.
- Portfolio evidence of learning achieved.

Summary

Chris has made a lot of progress in this chapter, and I hope that you have done so, too. Starting with a checklist of components that impact on learning in the workplace, Chris was able to choose a relevant workplace for scrutiny, and to rate it in a meaningful way that provided an opportunity for discussion and the reaching of a consensus with colleagues.

Awareness of loopholes is only useful if a way is provided to improve the situation, and Chris was able not only to differentiate and prioritise, but also to plan against specific and measurable targets.

In the early chapters of this book we examined the responsibility of supervisory managers to enable learning. The purpose of Chapters 7 to 10 has been to look carefully at workplaces themselves in terms of their capacity to support a learning culture. There is always a gap between the ideal and the achievable, but this should not prevent us from making an effort to make workplaces as good as they can be at supporting learning.

In the final chapter, I shall summarise the ideas that we have encountered throughout this book, and hope to convince you that attention to workplace learning will lead inevitably to improvement in the delivery of healthcare.

Chapter 11

Conclusions

Not too many years ago, the NHS was described in a *Guardian* article reporting on a House of Commons debate as being 'in a state of permanent revolution' (17 January 2001). If anything, the intensity of change since then has increased. Such seismic changes have economic, political, demographic and technological roots, and are part of the reason for the prevailing feelings of uncertainty among employees and service users. There are issues concerning recruitment and retention, resource allocation and planning that impact on day-to-day performance within the system. What is emerging as part of the philosophy underpinning these changes is an increased emphasis on governance and clinical quality to improve patient care, over and above the everyday concerns of efficient management. These have been fundamental drivers of the current reforms, and their influence on the cost and delivery of healthcare has been profound.

Debate about ways to increase resources for the NHS is partly, but not entirely, economic. People's values are a critical part of the debate, and it is possible to detect strong associations between these and the reforms that have been recommended. Expansion undoubtedly requires more resourcing, but modernisation also needs more qualified, better skilled and more flexible workers. Learning for all within the NHS is part of the process, so that these drivers (quality, efficiency, governance and patient care) are adequately understood and effective.

With the increasing pressure on the NHS to keep staff up to date, equipped with flexible and adaptable skills profiles, and with commitment to make a contribution over the long term, it is becoming necessary to look for creative ways to invest in people development. However, if this is confined to conventional solutions – taking people away from the workplace and sending them on training courses – the costs in financial and productivity terms will become increasingly prohibitive.

Recognition of the need for efficiency and cost-effectiveness, and growing understanding of the relevance of learning connected with work, have meant that it has become increasingly common to look to the workplace as an appropriate site for learning. Conventional 'training' is increasingly being complemented by innovative approaches to 'learning', often delivered via new and emerging technologies that seem to offer significant advantages in terms of ease of access. Learning that is concerned with performance can occur *for, at* and *through* work. Learning *for* work might include initial training, conferences and seminars – occasions that take people away from the workplace in order to learn. However, learning *at* and *through* work is generally the way that people learn and understand procedures, protocols and ideas that are relevant and significant in *order to do the job*.

The underlying economic environment

No organisation operates within a vacuum. External influences have a significant impact on decisions and emergent strategies, and these have a follow-on effect on day-to-day operations. Global events such as 9/11 and 7/7 eventually affect every organisation as it struggles to survive and prosper in shifting economic circumstances.

This is no less so in the public sector, where economic and socio-political conditions are inherited from past and present government actions. In the case of the NHS, like all public-sector bodies, national economic circumstances influence decisions about overall funding. In buoyant economic times more revenue is likely to be allocated to healthcare delivery and then by cascade to education and training for healthcare employees. The balance of revenue allocated to one economic sector – health rather than defence, for example – will vary from year to year, from regime to regime, and according to the political philosophy of the party in power.

In the NHS, change is a common occurrence which affects everyone to some extent – involving new technologies, increasing expectations, and the need to survive through a greater emphasis on the capability of the workforce. In response to these and other pressures the stated intention of the Government has, over the last five years, become more focused on health service delivery and the quality of the patient experience, and this has resulted in significantly increased spending between 2001 and 2007–08. Early indications are that this level of spending will not continue, and that from 2008 onward we will be expected to continue to deliver high-quality healthcare but at reduced cost.

Within the NHS there is considerable investment in recruitment and support for career progression through learning, and this has much wider resource implications than finance alone. Much attention has been given to changing the pattern of delivery via changes in structure – for example, the emergence and growth of primary care trusts (and now their predicted merging and possible demise), which currently hold the majority of the NHS budget. New forms of financial accountability are matched by greater flexibility of skills mixes and role accountability, and operationally via increased emphasis on governance and evidence-based practice. These changes have direct implications for the way in which work is done, and there is a strong requirement for increased awareness and understanding among NHS employees.

> Funding to support learning is governed by national and local circumstances which vary over time and which dictate the level and direction of investment made.

The policy context

The directions that are taken by policy decisions to support learning are often not made very explicit, and they vary across time. Throughout the twentieth century there has been a long and unedifying history of failed initiatives to promote education and training among the workforce in the UK. There has been a latent tension surrounding responsibility for the funding and provision of training. Should it be the Government that takes responsibility or should the employer drive the agenda? In some sectors we have witnessed training levies, training boards and the patchy growth and recognition of the value of NVQs. In the healthcare sector there has been little coherence and consistency across the various professional groups, with some groups (e.g. support staff, who represent more than 40% of the sector) missing out significantly on development opportunities. We are now seeing the adoption of a Knowledge and Skills Framework (KSF) that underpins an *Agenda for Change*. This is part of a continuum of past and future changes, and they dictate the direction that is to be followed by learning to support practice. The new White Paper on skills, *Getting on in Business, Getting on at Work* (published by the Department for Education and Skills in 2005) is just the latest in a long line of attempts to engage young people in appropriate vocational pathways by:

* tackling low participation by those over 16 years of age
* providing better vocational routes
* re-engaging those who are disaffected with learning.

Meanwhile, the recent White Paper from the Department of Health, *Creating a Patient-Led NHS* (published in 2005) tackles these issues from a completely different angle by inferring that the opening up of choice will force learning-led change.

In broad terms, the amount of funding available makes a difference to how much education and development can be provided. Funds have to be not only available but also accessible. The likelihood is that more funding will mean that more provision for learning will be made, there will be more awareness of opportunities, and more take-up will be identifiable. Equally, the increasing importance of qualifications as evidence of preparedness for work influences the direction that policy takes. More funding allows a greater variety of pathways and end-points (qualifications) to be offered. The rise in the significance of work-based and e-learning and the high priority given to new ideas, such as the recently lauded and then closed NHS University, are all examples of the direction that learning might take. However, ideas are often discarded as fast as they are taken up, and the field remains confused.

This speed of change may have something to do with the extent to which national initiatives transfer smoothly to local practice. For example, the extent to which the NVQ framework has become embedded is typical. There was a high level of expectation in the mid-1990s that NVQs would offer an innovative approach to the standardisation of skills training and the continuing development of those skills. The framework was intended to cover all levels – from those with Skills for Life needs to those with advanced practice experience – and thus all job specifications. However, take-up has been patchy from sector to sector, and even where it is well established, coverage is confined to the lowest levels, NVQ 1 and 2 having made the greatest impact. Rather than being delivered in the workplace as initially intended, and rather than being assessed via everyday practice, they are overwhelmingly delivered via simulation elsewhere. However, the greatest weakness of NVQs is the extent to which they recognise existing knowledge and skills, rather than offering a means of future development. Therefore, although they are better than no training at all, they do not fully serve the purpose for which they were intended.

Policy decisions are influenced by present Government initiatives and mandates, many of which have been inherited from previous regimes.

Socio-political trends

Political environments and social trends lead to expectations about how the workforce should be trained, deployed and rewarded. These decisions will be made at national level, but will be interpreted and implemented widely, both regionally and locally, with varying emphases and outcomes. The impact of international influences also has some bearing, even within a UK-centric organisation such as the NHS. European and US best practices are monitored and frequently taken into account at policy-making level. There are also variations across time. Whether education and training are seen as necessary has altered significantly in recent decades, and this influences decisions to provide as well as decisions to take part in work-related learning.

At the start of the twenty-first century we are perceived to be working in a 'knowledge economy' in the UK. The number of unskilled jobs is a fraction of what it was a decade ago, and the emphasis on education for the majority is now greater than ever before – witness the Government's stated intention to have more than 50% of young people studying at university by 2005. This has to be set beside the tensions of funding (think of the recent debate about top-up fees) and the latest media profiling of the lack of plumbers and electricians in the UK.

Changes in the public sector mean that the idea of a 'job for life' is no longer assumed, and flexibility and adaptability are required attributes for the modern healthcare worker. Social trends are towards several 'portfolio' careers that demand continual learning in support, and the claim that we live in a 'knowledge society' is rarely challenged. It is undoubtedly true that the complexity and skills levels required of NHS staff have grown exponentially during the last decade.

The Government's modernisation programme for the NHS (and for the public sector generally) aims to ensure a dynamic public sector where innovation is encouraged in pursuit of efficient and effective service provision. Learning and improvement go hand in hand.

> Social trends and the perceived value of training and learning will influence the emphasis that is placed on decisions to fund and otherwise support learning.

Individual learning processes

Expectations about learning are frequently coloured by early experiences at school. Whether these were good or bad, our memories about learning are likely to be vivid, and we can probably all recall uncomfortable situations and unpleasant incidents. Despite differences in background and experiences, we all nurture hopes and expectations about life, career and status. These varying life chances will influence our approach to learning and the investment of time and effort that we make. Equally, there will be social and lifestyle factors that influence our plans and actions with regard to the priority that we give to learning at any time.

People learn in a variety of ways, and it is apparent that some progress more easily than others. We have strengths in different areas – we might have musical ability, or we might be athletic, or we might be good at maths. So it is that some individuals will progress in guided, formal learning settings, whereas others are more autonomous, independent learners. Some are reflective and some are activist – some prefer to debate while some prefer to read a book as a means of learning. Some individuals have insight into their own learning style and some do not. Informal workplace learning will occur via a range of processes, and opportunities need to reflect this.

Much attention is given to learning styles. Useful as it is to know about our preferred style, the fact is that we all demonstrate a range of learning styles, albeit with strengths in one or more of them. The fact that our style can and will adapt to circumstances and needs is frequently overlooked.

It is less frequently acknowledged that the way we learn is influenced by the intended outcome. How often do we stop to ask ourselves why we are learning something? A task-related skill requires a different learning strategy to the understanding of a body of facts and figures. And they both differ from the strategy required to learn about managing workplace relationships. Over the years and with growing experience we develop automatic mechanisms to cope with different learning needs. The greater the opportunity there is to practise, the more refined this skill of 'learning to learn' will become.

Individuals demonstrate a range of expectations, mode, style and preference for level of formality while learning, and their interest and thus their rate of participation will vary accordingly.

The purpose of learning

Whether the purpose of learning is to improve skill, understand new concepts or broadly improve performance, organisational and individual plans may take different directions. Organisations habitually focus on competence as a means of assessing standard of ability to do the job, particularly with regard to workplace skills. Arguably this measures a generally agreed norm, or what an employee can do. However, this might not entirely concur with what an individual *does* do, and the difference is influenced by such things as disposition, environment, workload, support, and so on.

Some people enjoy learning for its own sake, and gain personal satisfaction from the sense of control and progress that this offers. This kind of learning may be skills or knowledge based, but is generally self-directed and self-managed. Much of this can take place informally at work. It is likely to be opportunistic (although it is sometimes planned by the individual him- or herself), is usually multi-faceted and is frequently ad hoc. Often it is not legitimised by the name of 'knowledge', but it is arguably the most pervasive and relevant form of work-related learning. Benefit can be gained by sharing such learning with colleagues. When teams share ideas this will lead to increased understanding, and ultimately this can result in considerable organisational change.

What prompts one person to want to learn will probably differ from the factors that motivate another. Recognition of this simple fact can lead to greater understanding of how people might be helped to recognise their individual drivers, and can thus lead to more efficient choices with regard to learning needs and solutions.

> Learning needs range from skills improvement to greater knowledge to a desire to enhance capability, all of which will lead to improved performance. They are all individual drivers for learning and can be accommodated through work.

Individual commitment to learning

It is generally accepted that the less opportunity a person has had for formal learning in the past, and the fewer formal qualifications they have gained, the lower their confidence level about current learning is likely to be. Equally, the lower the level of confidence, the less persistence is likely to be brought to the task of learning and the application of that learning. In other words, those who need to learn are likely to be the very same people who throw in the towel early. What can be done about this?

There is undoubtedly a group of workers who merely want to come to work, do the job and then go home again, and who have no desire to 'progress' through learning. Is there a place in the modern NHS for such people? In fact the NHS has changed so much over the last 10 years that anyone who has worked in any capacity in the service will have done some learning. No job is the same as it was, and I would defy any employee in healthcare to demonstrate that they do things the same way now as they did when they started. How could this be unless they have done some learning? This is progression, surely, and I would argue that we *do* need such people.

The extent to which an individual has a true and realistic perception of him- or herself as a person and as an employee (his or her 'self-efficacy') will influence his or her capacity to learn informally at work. This is part of a person's individual personality and psyche, and it is likely to emerge and strengthen with experience and maturity. This perhaps helps to explain why older learners are invariably successful, despite having had setbacks in their earlier learning career. Self-assessment and realistic goal setting are a product of individual reflective practice that articulates very closely with the ability to learn informally.

> Disposition to learn, self-confidence and persistence with learning will vary from individual to individual and will cause variations in the amount and form of informal learning that occurs.

Leadership and collaboration

The socially situated, experiential nature of learning as described in this book presents something of a challenge for many organisations. If learning is embedded in work, then it must occur in a highly decentralised fashion. What, then, is the role of the training and development function in trusts? Where are the boundaries between this group and the supervisory manager who is present and responsible on a day-to-day basis for the performance – and increasingly for the development – of individual skills?

Actually, this is not a zero sum game – it is not a question of 'either/or'. We find that the circle of people involved in supportive learning is widening, and where and how learning takes place is greatly expanded.

The role of the training function in providing outside (formal) knowledge is still vital, but processes that tap into individual and group knowledge can supplement and complement training courses. Guidance on the development of learning communities is needed and is often scarce. Collaboration and leadership between managers will ensure that all approaches are taken and blended towards a satisfactory learning outcome.

The role of the supervisor becomes more complex with every new factor that is taken into account – culture, trust, motivation and learning style all come into play, not just with regard to individuals but also in relation to groups. The supervisory manager is crucial in this respect, as they can inspire learning among staff in a variety of ways.

- They can attempt to create a positive climate for learning, to combat the feeling that it is intruding upon work.
- They can offer guidance on purpose, highlighting the links between learning activities and the trust's objectives.
- They can provide access to learning resources, external opportunities and people, including training and development specialists.
- They can help to create opportunities for employees to test out and consolidate their learning.
- They can provide regular and constructive feedback on learning and performance.

Regrettably, supervisory managers are not always assessed or assisted in their attempts to help learning at work. This raises the possibility of a serious knock-on effect on those who report to them, since the attitudes that these individuals absorb from their supervisors will most certainly shape their own approaches to learning.

Modernisation and health improvement

With spending on the NHS currently running at double the level that it was in 1997, the service still often appears to be struggling to maintain quality and high standards of provision. Modernisation has been undertaken at breakneck speed, and inevitably this has led to some destabilisation. A recent survey of more than 40 countries shows that for 15 years

England has gone furthest and fastest down the road of reform, with the intention of improving efficiency and cutting costs. In the short term this kind of activity is difficult to sustain, and it will inevitably have knock-on effects on the delivery of service.

In this book I have argued that we can counter the effects of such change by encouraging continual, non-formal, socially located learning. By working together and by learning and sharing our experiences, we can drive change rather than respond to changes that are imposed upon us.

Further reading

- Department for Education and Skills (2005) *Getting on in Business, Getting on at Work*. The Stationery Office, London; www.dfes.gov.uk/publications.
- Department of Health (2005) *Creating a Patient-Led NHS*. The Stationery Office, London; www.dh.gov.uk/publications.

Index